This book is written to appeal to both professionals and lay readers. Psychiatrists, nurses, and social workers do not like the label 'schizophrenic.' The label defines a person with schizophrenia as 'schizophrenic' and does not do justice to his or her humanity. Professionals do not need sociologists to tell them that the label is wrong-headed. As many in the field testify, people with schizophrenia have many qualities other than being 'schizophrenic.'

The book is also written to appeal to family members and friends, who need to understand, not just the disease entity, but also society's as well as their own reaction to it. A critique of the typical responses in society to schizophrenia and arguments for how it could be otherwise are needed.

Finally, the book is written to appeal to sociologists. Critical features of society and social life are disclosed in the examination of schizophrenia. The book draws selectively upon the work of George Herbert Mead, Kenneth Burke, Morris Rosenberg, Talcott Parsons, M.M. Bakhtin, and Max Weber to address the problems that surround the subject and treatment of schizophrenia ... From the sociological study of schizophrenia, we learn about what it means to be a human being. We learn about human character. Through the example of their suffering and survival of their affliction, people with schizophrenia teach us about ourselves and what it means to be a member of society.

From the Prologue

ISBN 0-8020-7830-3

9 780802 078308

SO-BVP-641

UNIVERSITY OF TORONTO PRESS

1995

Towards a Sociology of Schizophrenia
Humanistic Reflections

Schizophrenia, at one time considered by many clinicians to be a psychological response to oppressive upbringing, is now generally accepted as a physical illness. While Keith Doubt does not quarrel with this current view, he does challenge the positivistic assumptions that tend to accompany it. Throughout this fascinating survey of the literature on schizophrenia, Doubt presents a critique of society's neglect of those afflicted and promotes a humanistic understanding of them.

Doubt draws on several disciplines and uses the works of such diverse writers as Vygotsky, Piaget, Deleuze, Laing, and Torrey. While he rebukes medical practitioners for ignoring the social dimensions of schizophrenia, he is equally critical of postmodernism's tendency to valorize the mentally ill. Nor does he sympathize with particular sociological approaches which, he believes, emphasize society's reactions to the illness – often at the expense of the afflicted person. Thus, a major part of Doubt's project is to place the individual at the centre of sociological theorizing about schizophrenia.

This thought-provoking study offers an alternative perspective on schizophrenia to scholars and professionals, as well as to those who live with the disease. Doubt offers practical recommendations, which he hopes will bring relief to sufferers, and helpful insights to those engaged in treating or assisting people with schizophrenia.

KEITH DOUBT is an associate professor of sociology at Truman State University, Missouri.

Towards a Sociology of Schizophrenia

Humanistic Reflections

KEITH DOUBT

UNIVERSITY OF TORONTO PRESS
Toronto Buffalo London

ISBN 0-8020-0845-3 (cloth)
ISBN 0-8020-7830-3 (paper)

Printed on acid-free paper

Canadian Cataloguing in Publication Data

Doubt, Keith
    Towards a sociology of schizophrenia

    Includes index.
    ISBN 0-8020-0845-3 (bound)
    ISBN 0-8020-7830-3 (pbk.)

    1. Schizophrenia – Social aspects.   I. Title.

    RC514.D68 1996   362.2'6   C95-933004-6

Portions of chapter 1 were previously published as 'Mead's Theory of Self
and Schizophrenia' in *Social Science Journal* 29/3 (1992). Portions of chapter 2
were previously published as 'A Sociological Hermeneutics for Schizophrenic Language' in *Social Science Journal* 31/2 (1994) and 'A Burkean
Hermeneutics for Understanding the Social Character of Schizophrenic Language' in *Symbolic Interaction* 17/2 (1994). The extract in the Epilogue was
published as 'Volunteering' in *Schizophrenia Digest* 2/2 (1995). In chapter 4,
excerpts from *Dreamtigers* by Jorge Luis Borges, Copyright © 1984, renewed
1992, appear courtesy of the University of Texas Press.

University of Toronto Press acknowledges the financial assistance to its publishing program of the Canada Council and the Ontario Arts Council.

Contents

Acknowledgments

This book developed with the help and interest of several students, some of whose names I gratefully mention: Kaori Sato, Donna Foppe, Lori Wingate, Maureen Leonard, Patrick Granada, Angela Mayte, and Lynn Biberdorf.

Truman State University (formerly Northeast Missouri State University) supported this work with several faculty grants and a sabbatical leave.

I am indebted to the education I received in the Graduate Programme in Sociology at York University with Alan Blum and Peter McHugh.

I dedicate this book to the patients in the Social and Community Orientation Program (SCOP) at Queen Street Mental Health Centre, Toronto, Ontario, and the residents of Countryside Rehabilitation Center, Kirksville, Missouri, whom I have had the privilege to spend time with and get to know.

I thank Susan, Danielle, and Aprile for their love.

PROLOGUE

Towards a Humanistic Understanding

The redeeming power of reflection cannot be supplanted by the extension of technically exploitable knowledge.

— Jürgen Habermas[1]

This book undertakes a concerted examination of schizophrenia as a social phenomenon while supporting the medical understanding of schizophrenia as a biological illness. Schizophrenia is not, as popular culture sometimes understands it to be, the actually rare phenomenon of split personality; nor is it now viewed by clinical psychologists, as it once was by some, as a person's creative response to an untenable, oppressive family situation. Within the scientific community, schizophrenia, like Down's syndrome or Alzheimer's disease, is understood as a fact of nature, and this view, at the political and institutional level, is the hegemonic one.[2]

The clinical symptoms of schizophrenia are: altered senses, including exaggerated or diminished perceptions of sight, sound, touch, taste, and smell; inability to sort information and respond appropriately; loose mental associations that lead to confused trains of thought; delusions; visual and auditory hallucinations; an altered sense of self; and emotional and behavioural changes ranging from complete passivity to severe overreactions.[3]

Schizophrenia affects 1 per cent of the world's population. In

Canada, it is estimated that '270,000 will be diagnosed with schizophrenia at some point in their lives.'[4] There is uncertainty as to what exactly 'causes' schizophrenia, but within the research community there is certainty that schizophrenia is a physical rather than a social or psychoanalytic pathology. There is no known cure for schizophrenia, but antipsychotic medications can suppress (with varying degrees of success) the symptoms, at certain costs and risks to the patient.

The brain is a part of the natural world. The person afflicted with schizophrenia has a brain that is diagnosed as diseased. When dysfunctional (for instance, when there is an abnormal level of neurotransmitters in the brain), the human being suffers. Today medical science examines the genetic and neurological nature of the pathology to such a high and exclusive degree that the subject of how schizophrenia is socially defined is almost entirely neglected. 'Participation in the social system,' Talcott Parsons writes, 'is always potentially relevant to the state of illness, to its etiology and to the conditions of successful therapy.'[5] To acknowledge schizophrenia as a fact of nature does not preclude the subject from sociological examination.[6] While it is a biological illness, schizophrenia is also a social illness; it is subject to social understanding and influence. Parsons's statement suggests the need for a sociological examination and identifies the specific focus that such an examination ought to have.

'"Being sick" constitutes a social role'; it is not 'simply a state of fact' or a 'condition.'[7] Is there a viable sick role for people with schizophrenia? If not, why not? This study examines these questions. It also examines the roles that society ascribes to those with schizophrenia and asks how it could be otherwise. There is a pressing need to draw upon the rich resources and analytical skills of sociology to confront society's impoverished understanding of schizophrenia as a social phenomenon.

Previous studies have gone awry on this point. A sociology of schizophrenia which amounts to nothing more than a critique of the psychological profession is not really a sociology of schizophrenia. The approach of this book is atypical in that it does not dichotomize. The negative ways in which schizophrenia is responded to within the family and society are critical and consequential, but these negative interactions do not establish causal explanations of schizophrenia as a pathology. Unlike most social constructionists, I accept the neurological account of schizophrenia. At the same time, I resist the positivistic assumptions which undergird the neurological account. Medical science promises a cure for schizophrenia, but such a promise, in and of itself, does not address what schizophrenia is as a social phenomenon.

Human beings are organic things; human beings are more than organic things.[8] Human beings are agents with motives. Values are a resource for the action of human beings. Some believe that human beings have souls; that is, there is a non-empirical aspect of human nature. If these notions hold for our understanding of one another, why would they not hold for people with schizophrenia? The logic that governs the action of people with schizophrenia is not that of biological necessity; rather, it is a social logic. This logic is seldom recognized or appreciated.

The purpose of this book is to enlarge the social epistemology through which members of society, lay and professional, relate to people afflicted with schizophrenia. My approach is theoretical. At times, it is philosophical. The practical hope is that such reflections, grounded in examples from everyday life, will address constructively the problem of society's neglect and misunderstanding of the seriously mentally ill. To develop an enlightened understanding of schizophrenia is to provide those with schizophrenia better opportunities to participate more meaningfully and inclusively in the social world.

Society needs to do more than growl at the stone that hits the body of the human being with schizophrenia. Lament is understandable, but we can do more than that, if only for the sake of those afflicted. Pity creates self-pity, and many with schizophrenia have moved beyond the stage of self-pity.

The question of why certain people rather than others are struck by schizophrenia is not the only issue. The question of the effects on the human being struck is a parallel concern. To address the first is to engage in an empirical study. To address the second is to develop a humanistic perspective. This book does the latter.

This book is written to appeal to both professionals and lay readers. Psychiatrists, nurses, and social workers do not like the label 'schizophrenic.' The label defines a person with schizophrenia as 'schizophrenic' and does not do justice to his or her humanity. Professionals do not need sociologists to tell them that the label is wrong-headed. As many in the field testify, people with schizophrenia have many qualities other than being 'schizophrenic.'

The book is also written to appeal to family members, friends, and those afflicted, who need to understand, not just the disease entity, but also society's as well as their own reaction to it. A critique of the typical responses in society to schizophrenia and arguments for how it could be otherwise is needed.

Finally, the book is written to appeal to sociologists. Critical features of society and social life are disclosed in the examination of schizophrenia. The book draws selectively upon the work of George Herbert Mead, Kenneth Burke, Morris Rosenberg, Talcott Parsons, M.M. Bakhtin, and Max Weber to address the problems that surround the subject and treatment of schizophrenia. In chapter 4 a critique of the postmodern understanding of schizophrenia is provided. From the sociological study of schizophrenia, we learn about what it means to be a human being. We learn about human character. Through the example of their suffering and the survival of their affliction, people with schizophrenia teach us about ourselves and what it means to be a member of society.

Towards a Sociology of Schizophrenia:
Humanistic Reflections

1

SELF

George Herbert Mead

The brain is the source of everything that we are. It is the source
of everything that makes us human, humane, and unique. It is
the source of our ability to speak, to write, to think, to create, to
love, to laugh, to despair, and to hate.

– Nancy Andreason[1]

In *Surviving Schizophrenia: A Family Manual*, E. Fuller Torrey identifies a primary issue for any sociological study of social interactions between people afflicted with schizophrenia and people not
afflicted with schizophrenia:

Sympathy for those afflicted with schizophrenia is sparse because it is
difficult to put oneself in the place of the sufferer ... Those who are
afflicted act bizarrely, say strange things, withdraw from us, and may
even try to hurt us. They are no longer the same person – they are *mad*?
We don't understand why they say what they say and do what they do.[2]

To address this issue sociologically, it is fruitful to introduce the
social psychology of George Herbert Mead.[3] Mead argues that, as
social actors, we look at and understand ourselves from another
or society's point of view and guide our behaviour accordingly.
For successful communication and constructive understanding to

occur, we engage in 'taking the view of the other' or the view of 'the generalized other' which represents social convention.

Our capacity to empathize with people suffering from schizophrenia is 'sparse,' Torrey says, because we have trouble putting ourselves in their place.[4] 'They say strange things; they withdraw from us; they may even try to hurt us.' For those suffering from schizophrenia, the simplest tasks, such as using the telephone and buying milk, may be laborious struggles. More difficult tasks, such as building friendships and preserving intimacy, may be next to impossible. In addition, the lack of understanding shown by others, whether family members, strangers, or psychiatrists, greatly increases the difficulty of everyday living for people with schizophrenia. We are inclined not to see things from the perspective of someone suffering from schizophrenia and tend to deny him or her that social understanding that stems from human empathy. Consider the following example:

One patient, who believed he had a rat in his throat and asked the doctors to look at it, was told sardonically by the doctors that the rat was too far down to see. When the patient recovered he recalled that 'I would have been grateful if they had stated quite plainly that they did not believe that there was a rat in my throat.'[5]

To push the point, we seldom consider how people with schizophrenia show in their interactions with others the influence of another's perspective or 'the generalized other.' We tend not to recognize how people suffering from schizophrenia engage in social action even while psychotic because clinical psychology instructs us to see the cause of their behaviour as exclusively psychogenic.

John Strauss, a psychiatrist at Yale University and associate editor at *Schizophrenia Bulletin*, highlights this issue when he asks: 'Cannot a person's behaviour reflect both goal-directedness and pathology?'[6] Why does one perspective, the medical, preclude the other, the social? Why does the neurological point of view preclude the humanistic? Strauss continues:

My hypothesis is that the role of the person in mental disorder is not peripheral, merely as a passive victim of a disease to be fixed by medicine. Nor does my hypothesis agree with the view that the person and the disorder are the same, as is implied by much psychoanalytic theory. Rather, I propose that clinicians consider the person and the disorder as separable for the purposes of understanding both more adequately.[7]

Our topic is the self, not the body, of the person with schizophrenia, and how we might better recognize and understand the self of someone with schizophrenia.[8] Demonstrations of the argument are taken from two autobiographies, *Welcome, Silence*, by Carol North, and *Autobiography of a Schizophrenic Girl*, with Marguerite Sechehaye, and from Susan Sheehan's Pulitzer Prize–winning work *Is There No Place on Earth for Me?*, which carefully chronicles the tragic life of one actor with schizophrenia.[9]

Schizophrenia as the Invasion of Self

To start, we focus on Mead's commonplace remark 'We can distinguish very definitely between the self and the body.'[10] For instance, our body yawns because it may be tired or lacks oxygen or needs coffee, and our self stops the yawn so as to avoid offending the person with whom we are talking. Mead's simple but basic point transcends the monistic epistemology of positivism. In so far as social actors are reflective (to be a social actor is, by definition, to be reflective), social actors distinguish 'very definitely' between the body and self.

The questions in this context are: How can we distinguish 'very definitely' between the body and the self of the person with schizophrenia? Why is it that people tend not to make this distinction for the afflicted person? How might the person with schizophrenia respond to this neglect? How might this study locate ways of intervention into this situation?[11]

Consider Torrey's observation that 'schizophrenics' lose 'insightfulness':

Some people with schizophrenia are aware of the misfunctioning of their brain; this is what is called insight ... Such insight is usually lost as the disease becomes fully manifest. This is not surprising since it is the brain which is malfunctioning and it is also the brain which we use to think about ourselves. In fact I am always surprised at the many patients with schizophrenia who have insight.[12]

My goal is to reduce the surprise that even experts like Torrey have at the insightfulness of people with schizophrenia. It is important to secure ways to recognize the insightfulness of people with schizophrenia with respect to themselves, others, and their relations with others. How can we account for the fact that Torrey witnesses, but cannot explain, that people with schizophrenia have insight?[13]

In Susan Sheehan's *Is There No Place on Earth for Me?*, Sylvia is reported as saying to her mother: 'Ma, it's not me that's in here, it's the illness. The illness is stronger than I am.'[14] With this comment Sylvia is expressing her self, not her body, and her self's awareness of its victimization. 'In here' refers to Sylvia's body. When Sylvia says, 'It's not me in here, it's the illness,' she acknowledges the apparent displacement of her self as a consequence of her bodily affliction. Her body usurps her self, and the effect is that, within her own body, Sylvia feels homeless.

Sylvia's self, however, is not insignificant or unaware; nor is it non-existent. To be delusional, in Meadian terms, is to express a self as if that self were detached from one's body as well as the bodies and selves of those with whom one interacts.[15]

Mead says that 'we can lose parts of the body without any serious invasion of the self.'[16] For example, a person who loses a leg in a car accident may sustain a viable and lively self. The person may be unable to run, and running is a social activity; so perhaps I should qualify Mead's point by saying that, when a person loses a part of the body, the self may be psychologically compromised. But this compromise, Mead is saying, does not constitute a serious invasion of the self. When one loses a part of the body, the self may feel disoriented, depressed, or angry, but this loss of a part of the body is not a serious invasion of the self.

What, though, is the situation with schizophrenia? What is painful about watching people with schizophrenia struggle with their illness is that we see how the illness does constitute a serious invasion of the self. What is uniquely tragic about schizophrenia is that it confronts the character of the self, and thus the ability of the self to be itself. In *Autobiography of a Schizophrenic Girl*, we read:

... for horrible images assailed me, so vivid that I experienced actual physical sensation ... It seemed that my mouth was full of birds which I crunched between my teeth, and their feathers, their blood and broken bones were choking me. Or I saw people whom I had entombed in milk bottles, putrefying, and I was consuming their rotting cadavers. Or I was devouring the head of a cat which meanwhile gnawed at my vitals.[17]

Traditionally, sociological studies of mental illness have focused on how the various practices of families and social groups constitute a serious invasion of a member's self. The studies show how people with mental illness suffer the bad faith of others who have more power or status. Consider, for instance, Erving Goffman's 'The Moral Career of the Mental Patient' and his formulation of the betrayal funnel, or Harold Sampson and colleagues' 'Family Processes and Becoming a Mental Patient' and the pattern of accommodation, or Edwin Lemert's 'Paranoia and the Dynamics of Exclusion.'[18] Each study is excellent with respect to explicating how the social member *qua* deviant experiences a serious invasion of the self through a series of extremely negative social interactions, for example, the betrayal funnel, a pattern of family accommodation, or the dynamic of exclusion. People with mental illness unjustly lose their status as members of society.

This study differs by focusing on how schizophrenia, as a physical illness, constitutes a serious invasion of the self, which may then be what predisposes the afflicted person to society's labelling and abuse. When the self of someone with schizophrenia is preoccupied with the task of preserving self in the face of grotesque hallucinations and hostile voices, it cannot attend well to the task of interacting with others.

What does it mean, then, to say that schizophrenia constitutes a serious invasion of the self? In so far as the self is thus impaired, what is the nature of this impairment? Mead says that our body and our self do not share the same experience, that is, 'the body does not experience itself as a whole.'[19] While the loss of a part of one's body may limit the self with, say, anger, the loss itself does not impair the ability of the self to experience itself as a whole.

What, though, about the person with schizophrenia? What does it mean to say that schizophrenia constitutes a serious invasion of the self? The self of the person with schizophrenia may experience herself in the same way that the body experiences itself; that is, the self may be unable to experience itself as a whole. This accounts for why most neurological discussions of schizophrenia reason as if patients with schizophrenia have no self. To say that schizophrenia is a serious invasion of self, however, is not to say that the afflicted person loses self, that is, regresses to the state of a merely conscious animal who, in the words of Karl Marx, 'is one with its life activity.' The person with schizophrenia retains his self, that is, he continues to make his 'life activity itself an object of his will and consciousness.'[20]

Reflexiveness as a Survival Skill

Mead says that the chief characteristic of the self is that it is reflexive. The self becomes an object to itself, and by so doing, the self is able to experience itself as a whole. Susan Sheehan records her subject, Sylvia, as saying:

I have schizophrenia – cancer of the nerves. My body is overcrowded with nerves. This is going to win me the Nobel Prize for medicine. I don't consider myself schizophrenic anymore. There's no such thing as schizophrenia, there's only mental telepathy.[21]

How might we analyse the language in the preceding passage? We hear Sylvia's self attempt to compensate for its apparent displacement from the body. Sylvia's reflexiveness is fragmentary and contradictory. Sylvia seems hyper-reflexive; that is, her reflexiveness seems to fail to do exactly what it is that reflexiveness does for the self – namely, enable the self to experience itself as a whole.[22]

We imagine that the self of someone suffering from schizophrenia is in a state of panic when it experiences this impairment of its nature. Reflexiveness is to the self what walking is to the body. Just as not being able to walk disengages one from physical activity, losing the capacity to be reflexive disengages one from social interaction. The question thus becomes: What sort of wheelchair for the self does someone suffering schizophrenia need during a psychotic period?

In *Autobiography of a Schizophrenic Girl*, there is an example of the type of answer that we are looking for. Renee, a young girl with schizophrenia, comments on her interactions with her therapist:

What did me the most amazing good was her use of the third person in speaking of herself, 'Mama and Renee,' not 'I and you.' When by chance she used the first person, abruptly I no longer knew her, and I was angry that she had, by this error, broken my contact with her. So that when she said, 'You will see how together we shall fight against the System,' (what were 'I' and 'you'?) for me there was no reality. Only 'Mama,' 'Renee,' or, better still, 'the little personage,' contained reality, life, and affectivity.[23]

Notice how sensitive Renee's self is to another's language use: The third-person names, 'Mama and Renee,' rather than the abstruse, first-person pronouns, 'I and you,' facilitate the ability of Renee's self to identify with another, to take the attitude of the other, and so Renee's ability to achieve an affective, meaningful relation to another. Renee frequently mentions how important it was to feel connected to another during her illness and how difficult it was for her when she did not (whether because of the illness or because of the behaviour of other people).[24]

Self-Consciousness

People afflicted with schizophrenia have a self because people with schizophrenia exemplify self-consciousness. For Mead, self-consciousness has two connotations. One is rather complicated, referring to the ability to call out in ourselves a set of definite responses which belong to the others of the group.[25] The other is the recognition of one's body and bodily experiences as belonging to one's self. Let us consider the latter connotation first.

Until the rise of his self-consciousness in the process of social experience, the individual experiences his body – its feelings and sensations – merely as an immediate part of his environment, not as his own, not in terms of self-consciousness.[26]

Mead's description of the birth of a person's self-consciousness brings to mind an infant (whose self has yet to emerge) who has not yet discovered that its limbs are subject to its own control. We learn at an early age that certain motor functions are voluntary and subject to the will of our self. We are not, however, even as adults, always self-conscious in this regard. We may, for instance, tap our toes, bite our fingernails, or doodle while talking on the phone without being self-conscious of these physical activities. But imagine our confusion if we could not connect the experience of our body with the experience of our self. Say, for example, if we looked down at our hands and did not recognize their existence or acknowledge them as our own.

It is common for a person suffering schizophrenia to lose self-consciousness in this very manner. Consider the following account:

The arms and legs are apart and away from me and they go on their own ... I have to stop to find out whether my hand is in my pocket or not. I'm frightened to move or turn my head. Sometimes I let my arms roll to see where they will land.[27]

Here a person with schizophrenia lacks self-consciousness in the sense that self-consciousness involves the recognition of one's body as being one's own.

Here is why sexual activity for people with schizophrenia during a psychotic episode is awkward. While having sex, the afflicted person may not even be aware of his or her own body. The person may not recognize the body that is experiencing sex as his or her own body. To make the same point another way: Many suffering from schizophrenia are uninterested in sex in so far as they see that they lack that kind of self-consciousness that is, first of all, required to enjoy sex. This recognition is itself an exemplification of that second, more complicated, kind of self-consciousness to which Mead refers.[28]

The second type of self-consciousness, which is more difficult to account for, Mead describes as the ability to call out in ourselves a set of definite responses which belong to the others of the group; it is the ability to take the attitude of the generalized other in social interaction with other actors. 'But only by taking the attitude of the generalized other towards himself, in one or another of these ways, can he think at all.'[29] Taking the attitude of the generalized other towards oneself with others is the basis for meaningful communication in social discourse. When, therefore, we do not recognize someone suffering from schizophrenia as a self-conscious actor (someone capable of taking the attitude of the generalized other towards him- or herself [in whatever distorted and strange ways that self-consciousness may do so]), we lose the basis for meaningful communication with those suffering from schizophrenia. By drawing upon Mead's work, we can develop a stronger understanding of the person suffering from schizophrenia as a self-conscious actor. This development can lead to a greater degree of understanding between those afflicted and those not.

Torrey says that one of the earliest changes in the schizophrenic experience involves impairment in the process of empathy towards others. As the illness starts, 'the schizophrenic person loses the ability to put him/herself in the other person's place or to feel what the other person is feeling.'[30] Let us focus on the positive content of Torrey's point. Torrey says that the first evidence of schizophrenia is its effect on the self.

We are not born with a developed self; rather, it develops historically through social interaction. Schizophrenia usually appears in early adulthood, after a self has already developed.

What, then, happens to the self with the onslaught of schizophrenia? How does a self, which is already developed, cope with the invasion that is schizophrenia? What resources does the person possess to cope with and survive this onslaught? What resources are there other than the self? Does it not behoove us to address the self as an important variable for a better understanding of our subject?

Medication, which reduces and masks the symptoms of the illness, does not cure schizophrenia. While powerful medications allow the self to function more effectively, if not normally, in social interaction, overmedication can also hinder this ability. Medication is not a substitute for human understanding. People suffering from schizophrenia need empathy as much as medication. While the body of someone suffering from schizophrenia needs antipsychotic medication to suppress hallucinations and other symptoms, the self needs more. It needs understanding. To treat the body of someone with schizophrenia and to ignore the self is to do a disservice to the troubled and isolated individual.

Role-Taking

Mead says that a self becomes dormant and dysfunctional if one is either unable or unwilling to put oneself in the other's place.

It is through taking this role of the other that he is able to come back on himself and so direct his own process of communication. This taking the role of the other ... is not simply of passing importance ... The immediate effect of such role-taking lies in the control which the individual is able to exercise over his own response.[31]

In taking the role of the other, we are controlled by society, but, more important, we control our relation to society as well as society's relation to us.[32] If persons suffering from schizophrenia seem unable to take the role of the other, owing either to their illness or to others' view of them, it becomes difficult for them to control their relation to society as well as society's relation to them.

Carol North is one of a fortunate few whose schizophrenia was cured 'unexplainably' by kidney dialysis; since being cured, she has become a medical doctor and practising psychiatrist in St Louis, at Washington University. The title of her autobiography, *Welcome, Silence*, refers to the striking and wonderful experience of not hearing voices after many difficult and painful years.

'Something's different, really different.' 'What's different, Carol?' 'The silence.' 'The silence?' 'Yeah – it's, well, like, it's – deafening. The voices are gone. It's never been this quiet before.'[33]

Then North observes:

Life was so much easier now that I no longer toiled under the constant strain of monitoring all my thoughts every minute of the day to keep objectionable personal thoughts off the TV and radio.[34]

Welcome, Silence provides an insider's view of someone's self while psychotic. The first-person narrative reveals what Erving Goffman would call the 'back region' of the social actor while psychotic.[35] What we learn is that, while afflicted, the self of someone with schizophrenia is not that different from the self of someone without schizophrenia. From a dramaturgical perspective, North is completely normal. She had remarkable coping skills, and she was adept at covering the effects of her illness in her relations with family, friends, and psychiatrists.[36]

Gradually, I learned how to become a good actress, pretending that I was a normal person in spite of my symptoms. I recalled the cover-up skills I had developed back in childhood with Dr. Vandenberg's calendar and gold stars. Now I worked to apply and refine my old techniques. I learned to restrain myself from answering back or even looking around when the voices talked to me.[37]

It is worth mentioning who Dr Vandenberg is and explaining the reference to the calendar and gold stars. Dr Vandenberg was a therapist with a behaviourist perspective and one of the many care-givers who North saw when she first experienced her illness.

What did Dr Vandenberg recommend to North's mother for her child's unexplainable fear upon hearing voices and having hallucinations?

'I'll make a deal with you,' he said to me as he reached into one of his desk drawers. 'Here is a calendar for you to keep. Every day you're not afraid, your mom will put a gold star on that day. When you've earned thirty gold stars in a row, you'll get a bicycle.'[38]

It is interesting from a Meadian perspective to note what North learned, from this treatment; she learned, not only to conform to external demands and to others' expectations, but also to engage internally in the process of role-taking for the sake of her self's survival.

The next few nights I continued telling the truth about being scared, and the calendar remained empty. Finally I caught on. I was supposed to lie ... I was learning not to trust my own perception ... I learned never to tell anybody I was scared, no matter how scary things got.[39]

North discloses what is so difficult for someone suffering schizophrenia in social interaction: she engages in social interaction without being able to trust her perception of herself, others, or the world. In the absence of what Hegel calls 'sense-certainty,' North learns to trust her social ability, her ability to take the role of the other.[40] For North, this ability to take the role of the other is not compromised by the effects of her pathology, by her lack of conventionally sanctioned sense-certainty. If anything, her ability to take the role of the other is enhanced so as to compensate for the inability to take for granted that hers is a shared sense-certainty.[41]

The irony here is that what 'normals' trust in their interactions with people with schizophrenia is not their ability to take the role of the other, but their sense-certainty, namely, the perception of the other as 'crazy,' which leads to the labelling of the other as insane. 'Normals,' rather than take the role of the person with schizophrenia, depend upon their sense-perception that the other is insane. The irony here is that, from a sociological perspective, 'normals,' in their interactions with people afflicted with schizophrenia, are the weaker actors. Because the sense-certainty of someone suffering from schizophrenia differs so sharply from that of someone not suffering from schizophrenia, 'normals' are frightened by the difference. 'Normals' respond by 'labelling' the unhealthy member.

The afflicted member, however, is also frightened by how his or her self-certainty differs sharply from that of others. The afflicted member, at least in the first-person accounts of Renee and Carol, responds with the increased capacity to take the role of the other. This capacity becomes a survival tactic, a way to cope with one's affliction without 'going insane.' The tragedy here is that 'normals' do not help the afflicted person in this regard; that is, they do not help the afflicted person take the role of the other. Out of fear, 'normals' baulk and so fail to see the similarity between themselves and those afflicted with schizophrenia. 'Normals' fail to recognize how people with schizophrenia are like themselves in that people with schizophrenia are capable of taking another's role. 'Normals' fail to see and appreciate how people with schizophrenia are self-conscious actors.

Speaking further of role-taking and its importance to the individual, Mead says: 'The control of the action of the individual in a co-operative process can take place in the conduct of the individual himself if he can take the role of the other.'[42] To pursue this crucial idea, let us consider another, perhaps deeper, example of role-taking, quoted here at length, from *Autobiography of a Schizophrenic Girl*:

One day we were jumping rope at recess. Two little girls were turning a long rope while two others jumped in from either side to meet and cross over. When it came my turn and I saw my partner jump toward where we were to meet and cross over, I was seized with panic; I did not recognize her. Though I saw her as she was, still, it was not she. Standing at the other end of the rope, she had seemed smaller, but the nearer we approached each other, the taller she grew, the more she swelled in size.

I cried out, 'Stop, Alice, you look like a lion; you frighten me!' At the sound of the fear in my voice which I tried to dissemble under the guise of fooling, the game came to an abrupt halt. The girls looked at me, amazed, and said, 'You're silly – Alice, a lion? You don't know what you're talking about.'

Then the game began again. Once more my playmate became strangely transformed and, with an excited laugh, once more I cried out, 'Stop, Alice, I'm afraid of you; you're a lion!' But actually, I didn't see a lion at all: it was only an attempt to describe the enlarging image of my friend and the fact that I didn't recognize her.[43]

Notice the incredible coping skills Renee demonstrates in this passage. Renee is coping with the fact that her self cannot cope in this interaction or, more correctly, with the fact that her self lacks the perceptual stability required to cope in her interactions with her playmates. It is not that Renee's self is imperceptive (indeed, her self is extremely perceptive); it is that Renee's self lacks that particular and conditional sense-perception, the sense-perception of Alice as a recognizable person with stable, distinguishable features, that is taken for granted by the others with whom Renee is involved.

In terms of self, social perception, and social knowledge, Renee's situation is paradoxical, and yet it is typical of many first-person accounts of schizophrenia. On the one hand, Renee sees 'everything' (the people, the rope, the game, the rules, the timing of the interaction, the place, the expectation that others have of her) and yet recognizes nothing, that is, what is important – namely, the other person, Alice *qua* Alice. On the other hand, Renee sees nothing – namely, Alice *qua* Alice – and yet recognizes everything, for instance, the need of her self 'to cover' her incompetency in this situation and the need of her self to dissemble her perceptual difficulties with 'fooling' – 'actually, I didn't see a lion at all.'

As a self-conscious person, Renee recognizes her playmates' need for an explanation for her behaviour and complies with their need, not only for their sake, but also for her own. Renee is very much a social actor, and perhaps more of an accomplished actor than are her playmates.

Communication

Readers might wonder if this discussion exaggerates the healthy nature of a 'schizophrenic's' self in arguing that the human being suffering from schizophrenia retains a viable, albeit troubled, self during psychotic periods.[44] It is important to acknowledge this possibility, if only to show how it does not in any way undercut the irreplaceable usefulness of Mead's concepts for addressing the topic of self and schizophrenia.[45]

Mead's work focuses on the ways in which human language is different from the communication of animals, however sophisticated animal communication may be. Mead states:

> The importance of what we term 'communication' lies in the fact that it provides a form of behaviour in which the organism or the individual may become an object to himself. It is that sort of communication which we have been discussing – not communication in the sense of the cluck of the hen to the chickens, or the bark of a wolf to the pack, or the lowing of a cow, but communication in the sense of significant symbols, communication which is directed not only to others but also to the individual himself ... Of course, one may hear without listening; one may see things that he does not realize; do things that he is not really aware of. But it is where one does respond to that which he addresses to another and where that response of his own becomes a part of his conduct, where he not only hears himself but responds to himself, talks and replies to himself as truly as the other person replies to him, that we have behaviour in which the individuals become objects to themselves.[46]

During a psychotic period, the self of the afflicted person may seem to be so dormant that, from the viewpoint of the treating physician or the attending family member, the self is irrelevant to the understanding of this human being afflicted with schizophrenia. Here is where this study seeks to intervene with respect to how schizophrenia is socially defined, especially in the practices of the medical sciences.[47]

Consider the following report from *Autobiography of a Schizophrenic Girl* and how Mead's theorizing on the role of language in social observation helps us to appreciate Renee's astute observation of her own behaviour:

she did not comprehend my language, the language I used in talking to myself, comprising words discrete and unrelated and others self-created since I was denied the privilege of writing real words.[48]

And later:

I shed tears for hours, crying, 'Raite, Raite, was habe ich gemachte? (What have I done?), sorrowing in my own 'language,' in the meaningless, recurring syllables, 'icthiou, gao, itivare, giastow, ovede' and the like. In no way did I seek to create them; they came of themselves and by themselves meant nothing. Only the sound, the rhythm of the pronunciation had sense. Through them I lamented, pouring out the grueling grief and the interminable sadness in my heart. I could not use ordinary words, for my pain and sorrow had no real basis.[49]

Renee's self was unable to be itself in that she felt as if she could not communicate except like an animal. To Renee, and perhaps to others, her words became like a hen clucking, a wolf barking, or a cow lowing, and, as Renee says, her affliction would not allow her to do otherwise.

Notice Renee's comment at the end: 'I could not use ordinary words, for my pain and sorrow had no real basis.' Renee's pain and sorrow are real, but, in so far as she cannot communicate her pain and sorrow to others by allowing others to put themselves in her place so as to know what it is to be in her place, her pain and sorrow have no real basis, even to Renee herself. Thus her second pain, her social pain, is this schism between what she experiences and the absence of an adequate social knowledge of what she experiences. It is this second pain that sociologists can speak to because it is a pain for which the illness itself is not responsible. Rather, society is responsible.

To develop a viable and compelling sociology of schizophrenia, the subsequent chapters develop answers to the following set of questions: How do people with schizophrenia reflect while conversing with other selves? How can we comprehend this ability of people with schizophrenia? How do 'normals,' another label, reflect when interacting with 'schizophrenics'? In other words, how can we enlarge the social foundation, the normative epistemology of everyday life, to improve the lives and interpersonal relations of people who suffer from schizophrenia?

This book provides conceptual answers to these practical questions. It examines what Mead calls the 'conversation of gestures' that occurs between those afflicted with schizophrenia and those not. We can do more than growl at the stone that hits the body of the human being with schizophrenia. We can address the effects on the self of the person struck by this painful and disconcerting affliction. We can put ourselves in the place of the other.

2

LANGUAGE

Kenneth Burke

Intuition, leaping into the interior of morbid consciousness,
tries to see the pathological world with the eyes of the patient
himself: the truth it seeks is of the order not of objectivity, but of
intersubjectivity.

– Michel Foucault[1]

As seen in the previous chapter, one problem that exists for the
treatment and understanding of schizophrenia lies in the realm of
interpersonal communication. It is difficult for people with
schizophrenia to interpret others' language and behaviour and to
respond, not only appropriately, but also persuasively. The problem, moreover, is not one-sided. In the hospital setting, the language of people with schizophrenia is used to diagnose the
pathology, and, with this clinical goal in mind, the physician lis-
tens to the patient's language in a particular way, a way that may
not even hear the language as social or communicative. The physician hears the patient's language concretely – as a sign that corresponds directly and immediately with a pathology.

In this chapter, we examine the language of people afflicted
with schizophrenia, not as the sign of a pathology (although I do
not deny this aspect of the schizophrenic language), but as the
symbolic action of people who are self-conscious and intelligent.
To give human beings with schizophrenia the chance for more

inclusive relations with others, it is necessary to develop stronger positions from which to recognize and understand them as motive-guided actors. This requires looking at language. How do people with schizophrenia, even while psychotic, engage in symbolic action rather than behaviour that is externally governed? How do people with schizophrenia engage in action rather than motion?

The Social Character of Language

Much as we used Mead's work in the previous chapter to address self and schizophrenia, we use Kenneth Burke's work in this chapter to examine language and schizophrenia. Burke is an important social theorist and literary critic who influenced such sociologists as Erving Goffman, Hugh Duncan, Harold Garfinkel, C.W. Mills, Alan Blum, Peter McHugh, and even Talcott Parsons. Burke articulates a simple distinction between two fundamental types of meaning that he says is conveyed in all language used by human actors: One type of meaning, he calls 'semantic'; the other, he calls 'poetic.' Burke's formulation of the qualitatively different but nevertheless interrelated character of these two types of meaning encourages insightful interpretations of the symbolic character of language. While Burke's distinction is simple, his formulation of the relation between the two types of meaning is sophisticated. Burke argues that it is wrong to see the relation between these two types of meaning as antithetical and, at the same time, naïve not to see the relation between the two as dialectical.

Both types of meaning are ideal: Neither can exist independently of the other. Burke describes semantic meaning as

the ideal of the logical positivists. Logical positivism would *point* to events. It would attempt to describe events after the analogy of the chart (as a map could be said to describe America). And the significance of its pointing lies in the instructions implicit in the name.[2]

Burke argues that logical positivists have a non-dialectical understanding of how language is used by human actors in so far as logical positivists do not take into account the presence of the poetic type of meaning, which inevitably appears, even in the language of logical positivism. To make this point incisively, Burke observes the following irony:

We should also point out that, although the semantic ideal would eliminate the *attitudinal* ingredient from its vocabulary (seeking a vocabulary for events equally valid for use by friends, enemies, and the indifferent) the ideal is itself an attitude, hence never wholly attainable, since it could be complete only by the abolition of itself. To the logical positivist, logical positivism is a 'good' term, otherwise he would not attempt to advocate it by filling it out in all its ramifications.[3]

In contrast to semantic meaning, Burke says (and notice the difficulty in attempting to define poetic meaning, that is, to present poetic meaning in semantic terms):

Poetic meanings, then, cannot be disposed of on the true-or-false basis. Rather, they are related to one another like a set of concentric circles, of wider and wider scope. Those of wider diameter do not categorically eliminate those of narrower diameter. There is, rather, a progressive *encompassment*.[4]

Semantic and poetic meanings are notably different and yet profoundly interdependent. Such, for Burke, is the fundamental principle for the dynamic nature of symbolic action in social discourse.

Is the Meaning Semantic or Poetic?

To start the analysis, I introduce a series of everyday examples and 'fill out' their significance by recasting certain components of the examples so as to explicate the role of language in social discourse for those afflicted and those not.[5] In *Welcome, Silence*, there is the following exchange, which we have all experienced:

'Carol?' he asked. 'Are you Carol North?'

I nodded.

'Hi, I'm Dr. Hemmingway. ... 'What brought you here today?' he asked.

At first I thought he meant my car, but then he politely rephrased his query to ask what kind of problems I was having.[6]

When Dr Hemmingway, a psychiatrist whom North is meeting for the first time, asks: 'What brought you here today?' North cannot determine by herself whether the speaker means what mode of transportation brought her – a taxi, a car, a subway, a bus – or whether he means what specific problem – physical, social, or psychological – is the motive for her coming to see him. The question strikes North as ambiguous. Given the context, roles, and history, however, the question would not normally be heard as ambiguous. Hemmingway's expectation that the patient is coming to him for some sort of help is a variable that can be taken for granted by both actors. While North has grounds upon which to treat the question 'What brought you here today?' as ambiguous from a linguistic perspective, she has no such grounds from the perspective of the interaction itself. When North hears the question in isolation, as if it were unrelated to the rest of the interaction, she has trouble understanding and responding.

'What brought you here today?' has poetic potential. The question, while not a metaphor, tempts one with a metaphorical understanding. A car does not bring someone to some place because a car is not an active agent; it is a thing. It is the person driving the car who brings someone to some place. Things, which is what 'what' rather than 'who' asks for, are, to speak semantically, incapable of bringing someone anywhere. Our language and culture, however, are full of tales about things – trains, cars, boats – with personalities that bring and take people here or there. We understand and appreciate these stories according to their symbolic, rather than literal, meaningfulness.

North heard Dr Hemmingway's question as a fragment that was unrelated to the context in which it was asked; North was stymied by the question's figurative potential. Only after hearing a rephrasing that eliminated the poetic potential of the question was North able to respond. There was confusion with respect to whether another's language was governed by a semantic or poetic meaningfulness.

Here is another example of the same problem: In a TV documentary titled *48 Hours – Out of Mind*, the following exchange takes place with a homeless person who is diagnosed with schizophrenia: The interviewer asks, 'What's it like being on the street?' The subject replies, 'I don't even call this "on the street". Those cars are on the street. This is on the sidewalk. That term "on the street" is nuts!' Notice how the subject rebuffs the interviewer's question by exaggerating the absence of semantic precision in the phrase 'on the street.' (A common ploy among positivists.) The subject stresses that, speaking literally, he lives on the sidewalk. 'Those cars are on the street.' He is not a car. The subject transforms the phrase 'on the street' into a metaphor that lacks semantic intelligibility. This move stymies the interviewer.

The objection to the phrase 'on the street' is admittedly atypical, but, along the same line, consider the word 'skyscraper,' a dead metaphor because we typically do not reflect upon the word's poetic meaningfulness. Tall buildings do not scrape the sky. That word 'skyscraper' is nuts!

The socially determined intelligibility of the phrase 'on the street' and the word 'skyscraper' is grounded in what Harry Stack Sullivan refers to as 'consensual validation.'[7] According to Sullivan, the function of language is to serve as the handmaid of this consensual validation established by what Mead calls 'the generalized other.' By way of contrast, the beauty and charm of language for Burke is that there is more involved 'in linguistic processes and language symbols' than consensual validation, and Burke is adamant on this point.

Sullivan explains the logic of society's reaction to the language of people with schizophrenia this way: people with schizophrenia speak outside the realm of consensual validation and are therefore treated as pariahs.[8] Sullivan, however, says little with respect to the social character of schizophrenic language. For a critical sociology, consensual validation in and of itself is not the legitimating principle of social knowledge. While, yes, society rewards those who speak within the bounds of consensual validation and punishes those who do not, the task of a critical sociology is to understand these normative expectations, their limits, and how it might be otherwise.

Let us consider another example. In *Autobiography of a Schizophrenic Girl*, Marguerite Sechehaye reports Renee's relation to language as a self-conscious actor. As before, Renee's account depicts tension between semantic and poetic meaning, but from the opposite point of view of Carol North in *Welcome, Silence*.

What remained longest and was difficult to eliminate was the habit I had of saying, 'I am afraid of the wolf,' or 'of Die Polizei' (the police), words I uttered whenever I dreaded something or was in great distress. Actually when I said, 'I am afraid of the wolf' or 'of the Police,' I did not imagine either a wolf or the police for I was afraid of neither one nor the other. Therefore when people wanted to quiet me, asserting that there was no wolf and that they would protect me from the police, I was not at all reassured. The 'wolf' was something large and black, crying, 'hou, hou,' and gave rise to anxiety. But I neither saw nor thought of a wolf. Mama alone understood the diffuse panic hidden behind these phrases drained of sense and symbolism. She comforted me, saying, 'Why are you so afraid, nothing is going to happen to you; Mama is here to watch. Did you think of something that frightened you?' And most of the time she was right; I had thought for an instant that Mama might die; then I had forgotten the thought, the disquiet remained. Mama's question defined the idea generating the anxiety; then the anxiety itself disappeared.[9]

Renee is providing an explanation for her use of language, language that is most likely interpreted as delusional. For Renee 'wolf' and 'police' are metaphors, symbols that she uses to make meaningful the fear that she experiences as a result of her hallucinations. It was impossible for Renee to explain what caused her fear semantically; semantically, it was simply large and dark. Describing with symbols what scared her is a natural course of action for a 'symbol-using, symbol-making, and symbol-misusing animal.'[10]

The interactional problem that occurred was that people heard

Renee's metaphors, not as symbols, but as signs that were meant to correspond directly and immediately to what she was experiencing. Renee, however, did not see a wolf and she was not even afraid of a wolf; she was, though, afraid of what the wolf as a symbol referred to. When people responded to her by saying that they did not see a wolf, and therefore there was nothing for Renee to be afraid of, people told Renee nothing that she did not already know and only acerbated her isolation and pain. People failed to acknowledge that there was something real that made Renee anxious.

'Mama,' Renee's name for Sechehaye, her psychiatrist, showed more understanding of Renee's language. Mama did not treat Renee's language as meaningless 'code.' Mama allowed for the possibility that Renee's language was governed by a poetic sensibility. 'Wolf' and 'police' did not name that to which Renee was referring but 'encompassed' it.

Unlabelled Metaphors

Renee is isolated by her listener's non-recognition of her ability to speak with symbols. Renee's metaphors, wolf and police, are what Gregory Bateson would call 'unlabelled metaphors.'[11] An unlabelled metaphor is one for which there seems to be no intelligible grounding in something like the history of the patient, the social environment, culture, empirical reality, or reason.[12]

The term 'unlabelled metaphor,' however, is a gloss; the term does not by itself differentiate between the poetic meaningfulness of a schizophrenic's language and that of a non-schizophrenic. When someone not afflicted with schizophrenia uses an unlabelled metaphor, the listener trusts that there exists a semantic element that underpins the unlabelled metaphor. The listener either asks for clarification ('What do you mean?') or simply tolerates the confusion out of politeness. By way of contrast, when someone with schizophrenia uses an unlabelled metaphor, the listener distrusts that there is any semantic element undergirding the language. The person is judged crazy.

There are two ways to resist Bateson's concept. One is to cite an example in which there is a legitimate and socially sanctioned place for what Bateson calls 'unlabelled metaphors.' Consider the popular nursery rhyme 'Hey, diddle, diddle / The cat and the fiddle / The cow jumped over the moon / The little dog laughed to see such sport / And the dish ran away with the spoon.' Is there a labelled metaphor in this rhyme? Is not the pleasure (or displeasure for some) of the nursery rhyme its presentation of a series of unlabelled metaphors? The child identifies with 'the little dog [that] laughed to see such sport,' where the sport is the rhyme's purely poetic, that is, purely non-semantic, use of language. The semantic meaning of the rhyme, in so far as there is one, is that no semantic meaning is intended. Does this use of unlabelled metaphor render the rhyme uncommunicative or asocial?

For an adult version of the same point, consider the popular radio comedy 'Dr Science,' broadcast every day on National Public Radio. Why do people laugh at 'Dr Science' but look perplexed and even fearful, while listening to a 'schizophrenic's word-salad'? The humour of 'Dr Science' cleverly simulates bizarre paradigm shifts, craziness, disorderly thought, bogus logic, and unintelligibility. The humor of the radio program plays upon the possibility of talk being devoid of meaning. However, in so far as the audience, laughs and enjoys the narrator's talk, there is meaningfulness and social understanding.

For readers unfamiliar with the radio comedy 'Dr Science,' here is a short excerpt:

Dear Dr Science: What exactly are CDs made of? How do they get all that music on one small disc?

DR SCIENCE: All CDs are actually recycled LPs. These are pressed at huge plants just across the Mexican border. One plant spends all its time taking scratched copies of Carole King's *Tapestry* album and pressing them into Sinéad O'Connor CDs.

A second way to resist Bateson's concept of the 'unlabelled metaphor' as an apt description of schizophrenic language is to show how the metaphors that people with schizophrenia use are not as unlabelled as Bateson would have us think. Consider the following exchange in a video titled *Into Madness* produced by Alan and Susan Raymond in 1989. The video portrays relationships between families and siblings afflicted with schizophrenia. A father queries his son, Bob, diagnosed with schizophrenia: 'You don't like to take the pills? You think you could even get much better if you don't take medicine.' The son responds, 'It just depends on how I can hit the golf ball.'

The father's comments and question are difficult, not only for Bob, but also for the treating physicians. There is no known cure for schizophrenia, but antipsychotic medications can suppress the symptoms of schizophrenia, at certain costs and risks to the patient.[13] As Bob indicates, with respect to taking antipsychotic medicine, sometimes the ball goes straight down the fairway, sometimes it slices into the woods, and sometimes it just falls off the tee. Bob's metaphor is an excellent one, and hardly unlabelled, except from the viewpoint of a non-understanding listener.

On the Hegemony of Semantic Meaningfulness

In a clinical setting, to test the degree of thought distortion that a person with schizophrenia is experiencing, a physician asks the patient to explain 'the meaning of proverbs, which require an ability to abstract, to move from the specific to the general.'[14] In Burke's terms, the physician asks the patient to formulate the poetic meaning of proverbs like 'People who live in glass houses shouldn't throw stones,' 'Don't cross the bridge until you get to it,' or 'A rolling stone collects no moss.' The proverb is a proverb in that its poetic meaning, which is symbolically understood, is the essential meaning of the proverb. The proverb's semantic meaning is the inessential meaning. The test measures the hermeneutical skills of the patient and allows the physician to diagnose such symptoms as 'concreteness,' 'disconnectedness,' 'loosening of associations,' 'impairment of logic,' 'thought blocking,' and 'clanging association.'

There is a range of appropriate responses that demonstrate what a proverb like 'People who live in glass houses shouldn't throw stones' means, but, while there are several acceptable variations of an appropriate answer, there is not a limitless or random set of possibilities. That is, although we cannot precisely 'name' the measure that sanctions an appropriate response to this test (except to say that the response 'encompasses' the sense of the proverb), physicians nevertheless judge which answers from the patient are acceptable and which are not. Physicians employ what Harold Garfinkel empirically describes in *Studies in Ethnomethodology* as 'the documentary method of interpretation.'[15]

Typically, and somewhat ironically, the patient gives an answer that struggles with the semantic rather than the poetic meaning of the proverb, and in this fashion evades the task of providing for the proverb's poetic meaning. Physicians call this 'concreteness.' For example, in response to the demand to interpret the proverb 'People who live in glass houses shouldn't throw stones,' one patient replies, 'Because they might be put out for the winter.'[16] If this answer were given by someone playing the role of a 'wiseguy' or 'knocker,' the answer would represent a joke.[17] The answer undercuts the demand for compliance with a task whose everyday nature is poetic but whose clinical orientation is semantic. In so far as it is a literal response, the answer bypasses the physician's demand and becomes itself poetic. The answer transcends the demand to establish a shared agreement.[18] This is not to say that the patient who gave this answer is knowingly making a joke, being ironic, or satirical; rather, it is to say that the physician, given his or her goal of diagnostic accuracy, hears the subject's answer in a reductionist way. The physician does not hear the answer as a social one.

In the clinical setting, there seems to be little reflection on the problematic context of examiners' questions and subjects' answers. For instance, what is it to ask someone, whether mentally ill or not, the following set of questions?

Why does the wind blow? Why is your hair fair? Why does the sun come up in the morning? How does a fish live in water? Why did the man fall down in the street? How does your body make a shadow? Why are you alive? Why are you good?[19]

What do these questions, which seek to test a person's skills at conceptual formation, have in common? What language game is the patient being asked to play? What criteria does the experimental psychologist use to measure a successful as opposed to an unsuccessful achievement in this game? As a response to 'Why is your hair fair?,' why is 'Because I inherited it from my parents' a healthy answer and 'Because of something else; it's on my head; it comes from my mother' an unhealthy answer? What criterion legitimates the first and disqualifies the second?

The criterion is the normative preference for semantic meaning, which privileges clarity, precision, and naming as what demonstrates linguistic competence. This criterion suppresses a superior notion. Linguistic competence is not the privileging of semantic meaningfulness over and above poetic meaningfulness; linguistic competence is the awareness of the difference between semantic and poetic meaningfulness and an appreciation of the interplay between the two. The beauty and charm of language resides, not in the exchange of clear communication, but in the complex use of symbols to convey meaningfulness and achieve relation.

Most social scientists endorse the normative preference for semantic meaningfulness over and above poetic meaningfulness, especially in interactions with people afflicted with schizophrenia. For instance, Roy Wolcott writes:

Most of us, myself included, feel that people should talk straight and talk so that others can easily understand them ... most people would agree that ordinary language is more efficient, more logical, and more conducive to linguistic competence than schizophrenese ... I would suggest that the psychiatrist should seek to get the patient ultimately to use ordinary language.[20]

To talk straight is to talk where the standard of semantic meaningfulness dominates and, in a certain way, tyrannizes talk. Wolcott advocates that psychiatrists use behaviour modification to influence people with schizophrenia to comply with the normative order that favours talking straight rather than, say, poetically, humorously, satirically, ironically, and so on.

In her recent book *The Dinosaur Man*, Susan Baur shows much insight in identifying the problem which Wolcott uncritically promotes:

When I told the ward psychologist that Dallas Grey was letting me in on 'the code' that signaled for him the onset of torture, it was suggested that I tell him, 'We don't speak code in this hospital. When you're ready to talk my language, I'm ready to listen.' This was intended to teach Mr. Grey that crazy talk drives people away – a useful lesson.[21]

To tell the patient 'We don't speak code in this hospital' is to tell the patient that we respond only to language that is semantically governed. Language that is poetically governed, 'code,' is, according to the ward psychologist, inappropriate in the hospital setting and in society at large.

Baur goes on to describe many of the issues under discussion here. Consider the following account:

the day after Mr. Nouvelle had watched the Super Bowl on TV, I agreed with him that he was a lucky man to have been invited by the bouncing, big-bosomed cheerleaders to walk onto the field and feel their zucchinis. Such an honor must have made him feel good.

'No, it was not good,' he replied, annoyed by my response. 'You know there aren't any real women in a television set, just glass and a picture tube, so it feels cold.'

'Not very satisfying?' I asked, veering sharply to keep in step with his feelings but pleased to have him pop into my world.

'Well ... I could hold out my hand and feel their zucchinis.' And here he left my world as suddenly as he had entered it and traveled back in his 'photographic imagination' to the brilliant football field where dancing rows of cheerleaders leapt and spread their legs with obvious invitation. 'But,' he murmured, now deep within his dream, 'they put ice cubes in their underpants.'[22]

It is easy to map the course of this exchange between the patient and the therapist with respect to semantic and poetic meaning. The therapist takes the patient's delusional talk 'seriously'; she treats the talk as communicative and social by accepting it for its poetic meaning. When Mr Nouvelle senses what his therapist is doing, he replies at a semantic level. 'You know there aren't any real women in a television set, just glass and a picture tube.' The therapist now hears the patient entering 'her world' in response to her attempt to enter 'his world.' Moreover, she sees that she provoked his reaction. When she responds to him as now residing in 'her world,' which sanctions semantic meaning over poetic, the patient quickly returns to 'his world' that seems to prefer poetic meaning over semantic.

Baur's own interpretation of this exchange reinforces this Burkean analysis:

I did not have to be outsmarted by Mr. Nouvelle too many times before I dropped the interpretation of his delusions as my primary goal. For one thing, interpretation had connotations of accuracy that I found uncomfortable. For another, it didn't work. Even when I felt quite sure I had touched on the real significance of Coke, for example, Mr. Nouvelle would rearrange his world just enough to prove me wrong. He drove me to conclude that delusions cannot function as a protective shield unless they remain impenetrable. So I substituted participation as my objective, and without quite realizing it became more interested in the transactions that went on between speaker and listener – such as being shut out or being asked to applaud – than in correct interpretation.[23]

Baur recognizes that a dogmatic commitment to semantic understanding is both wrong-headed and ineffective when interacting with people with schizophrenia. Baur knows that participation in the transaction is where the action is. At the same time, participation is not gained upon the sacrifice of understanding; participation itself leads to understanding because participation is meaningful and significant in so far as it represents the course of symbolic interaction.

Baur's book is a testimony to the notion that we need to find better ways to establish interpersonal relations with people with schizophrenia, but Baur does not formulate the basis for her own success. For instance, in the exchange quoted above, Baur does

not seem to appreciate how Mr Nouvelle's final remark, 'But ...
they put ice cubes in their underpants' is a poetic response to her
earlier question, 'Not very satisfying?' The patient, unbeknownst
to the therapist, keeps the conversation going, albeit in a fashion
that the therapist had neither expected nor hoped for. The patient is in tune with the other. The patient even implicates
the other with respect to the intimacy between himself and his
therapist.

The interpretation of these and other interactions that I favour
is that, when a person with schizophrenia responds to another's
language that is either poetically or semantically lopsided, the
response becomes awkward and problematic. Sometimes, the
response looks like a 'reaction formation' to the 'lopsidedness' of
the other's language.[24]

Let me give an example. In the documentary titled *Frontline:
Broken Minds* aired on PBS, there is the following exchange with
Marge, a twin afflicted with schizophrenia.

MARGE: I'm not a committed and totally insane patient. I have a problem
and it has to be fixed where it can be and that's all the material.

INTERVIEWER: What will fix it?

MARGE: I don't know. I don't know. Like they said I might have to do
chemotherapy with instruments – electronic instruments with high voltage on it.

Given the nature of research on schizophrenia, to ask someone
with schizophrenia 'What will fix it?' is thoughtless. How could
Marge answer such a grandiose question in a reasonable and
appropriate manner? The interviewer shows no reflexivity.
Marge's parody of a semantically acceptable answer and its
absurdity is a 'reaction formation' to the absurdity of the interviewer's asking her this question. The point is that Marge's
response to the interviewer's lopsidedly semantically oriented
question ('Just get the facts') is as much a response to the thought-
lessness of the interviewer as it is an expression of her pathology.
'They said I might have to do chemotherapy with instruments –

electronic instruments with high voltage on it.' What did the interviewer expect to hear?

Metacommunication

Are people with schizophrenia capable of metacommunication? The answer is often, no. The classical statement on this issue is Gregory Bateson's. Bateson argues that schizophrenia is produced in a family setting in which a child experiences pathological communication from his or her parents. 'If you do x, you will be punished; if you do not do x, you will be punished.' To experience repeatedly and inescapably these double messages with nihilistic foundations leads to the development of a 'weak ego function,' which means the inability to discriminate 'communicational modes either within the self or between the self and others.'[25] The symptomology takes the following form: 'The schizophrenic feels so terribly on the spot at all times that he habitually responds with a defensive insistence on the literal level when it is quite inappropriate, e.g., when someone is joking.'[26] The reverse can also occur – the person responds metaphorically to a literal question so metaphorically that the response is characterized as delusional.

The question of whether people with schizophrenia are capable of metacommunication is as much sociological as it is neurological, linguistic, or psychological. The answer I support is that, like people in general, some suffering from schizophrenia are capable of metacommunication and some are not. There is much evidence from everyday interactions to show that people with schizophrenia are often quite competent with respect to metacommunication; one might even argue that, like many socially oppressed actors (think here of women and minorities), persons with schizophrenia are more aware of the metacommunication in a social interaction than is the oppressing, 'normal' member.

It is painful to watch a person suffering from schizophrenia being interviewed on a TV or video documentary because the afflicted member seems more in tune to the metacommunication of the interaction than does the interviewer. The afflicted member

seems sensitive, if not overly sensitive, to the banality of the interviewer's questions, the hidden agenda underneath the interviewer's 'pseudo-*Gemeinshaft*,' the contravening effect of the
observing camera, the ill-timed interruptions, the sympathetic but
unrealistic assumptions in the interviewer's questions, and so
on.[27]

The clearest context in which to think about whether people
with schizophrenia are capable of metacommunication is within
the context of art. One feature of 'outsider art,' art by people diagnosed as insane, is that it is an expression of the artist's experiences as a human being, sometimes a human being with
schizophrenia. This art is no less authoritative *qua* art than any
other art. Martin Ramirez, for instance, is a well-known artist
who expresses in his art his experiences as a human being with
schizophrenia.[28]

Unlike Bateson, R.D. Laing acknowledges the sensitivity of
people with schizophrenia to the metacommunication of a social
interaction and (romantically) sees this sensitivity as so superior
to a non-schizophrenic's that the language of people with schizophrenia is tantamount to high-minded mockery and clever parody, which almost always goes undetected by people not afflicted
with schizophrenia.[29]

Torrey recommends that all of Laing's writing on schizophrenia
be discarded as utterly preposterous and intellectually criminal,
but surely the humanism in Laing's work, however misapplied, is
something that must not be discarded.[30] When examining schizophrenia, Laing himself does not dichotomize when, for example,
he writes:

It should be noted that I am not here objecting to the use of mechanical
or biological analogies as such, nor indeed to the intentional act of see-
ing man as a complex machine or as an animal. My thesis is limited to
the contention that the theory of man as person loses its way if it falls
into an account of man as a machine or man as an organismic system of
it-processes.[31]

I do not claim here to have a method for reading the minds of people with schizophrenia (as if anyone had a method for reading another's mind). Nor do I claim that there is no foundation for differentiating the language of people with schizophrenia from the language of 'normals.' I do claim, however, that there is a social foundation for understanding the nature of schizophrenic language, and this matter deserves sociological study.

The basis for the pariah status of people with schizophrenia is as much the normal's misunderstanding of people with schizophrenic as it is the actual behaviour of people with schizophrenia. The interactions between people with schizophrenia and 'normals' are social. Society cannot realize its interest in rehabilitating this sadly misunderstood and alienated population without an effective hermeneutics to interpret the social basis of these interactions. Burke's work on the symbolic use of language by all human actors points to positive and constructive ways to develop such positions. It is time to shatter the interactional problem that the sociologist Morris Rosenberg thoroughly but uncritically describes as 'role-taking' failure.[32]

3

ROLE-TAKING

Morris Rosenberg and Lev Vygotsky

The justification for our concern about schizophrenic people
neither requires nor entails any assumptions about 'how the
schizophrenic's mind works': it partakes rather of judgements
that we make about each other (about suffering, for example)
from within the narrative enterprise of human lives.

– Peter Barham[1]

'Being Sane in Insane Places' Reconsidered

To develop a sociology of schizophrenia, it is necessary to critique previous sociological studies of schizophrenia. David
Rosenhan's 'Being Sane in Insane Places' is well known for
exposing the inhumane treatment of patients in mental hospitals
and drawing attention to the inadequacy of admission interviews
employed by psychiatric hospitals. The study's pseudo-patients
gained admission to mental hospitals by feigning one tell-tale
symptom of schizophrenia; they were not detected by hospital
staff during either the admissions interview or their subsequent
hospital stay.

To dramatize this point, Rosenhan writes: 'Despite the public
"show" of sanity, the pseudopatients were *never* detected.'[2] Three
paragraphs later, he adds: 'It was quite common for patients to
"detect" the pseudopatients' sanity.'[3]

What is happening here? First, Rosenhan says that the pseudo-patients were 'never' detected – a categorical remark. Then, Rosenhan says that the pseudo-patients were detected – they were detected by the patients in the hospital.[4] Is the detection by patients of no consequence? Why are the patients being denied the status of significant observers when, in fact, they are significant observers?

In his writing behaviour (and writing is behaviour), Rosenhan treats the patients as what Erving Goffman calls 'nonpersons' – 'Those who play this role are present during the interaction but in some respects do not take the role either of performer or of audience.'[5] This treatment is common for people with schizophrenia. Rosenhan unwittingly reinforces the prejudice that people with mental illness, in particular, those with schizophrenia, are incapable of taking the role of another. Rosenhan's study (which is itself a critique of this very prejudice) discloses the ubiquitous nature of society's bias towards mental illness.

Rosenhan's purpose is to critique the inhumane practices of psychiatrists and staff in mental hospitals. Rosenhan himself argues for a more compassionate perspective in the treatment of mental illness:

If patients were powerful rather than powerless, if they were viewed as interesting individuals rather than diagnostic entities, if they were socially significant rather than social lepers, if their anguish truly and wholly compelled our sympathies and concerns, would we not *seek* contact with them?[6]

Rosenhan's writing, however, belies his purpose. His desire to belittle the competence of the psychological profession is so strong that he exploits the stigma of people with mental illness. If people with mental illness detected the pseudo-patients in the hospital, why did not highly trained and educated doctors?

Rosenhan's sophistry prevents him from recognizing the significance of his unexpected finding – namely, that people with mental illness are capable of putting themselves in the place of others so as to understand the action of others. This point is crucial to the development of a sociology of schizophrenia. When people with schizophrenia are not recognized as capable of taking the role of others, they are excluded from the benefits of role-taking.[7]

The Unread Mind

Drawing upon the work of George Herbert Mead, Morris Rosenberg argues that insanity is socially constructed. Insanity, he says, stems from the failure of the 'normal' member to take the role of the 'psychotic' member.[8]

Let us consider an example of role-taking failure. In *Surviving Schizophrenia*, Torrey cites a person with schizophrenia who wrote: 'I believe we will soon achieve world peace. But I'm still on the lamb.' Torrey interprets the text this way:

He had confused lamb associated with peace with the expression 'on the lam,' the correct spelling of which he apparently did not know. There is no logical association between 'lamb' and 'lam' except for their similar sound; such associations are referred to as clang associations.[9]

Torrey interprets the talk as meaningless because, as Rosenberg puts it, the 'external observers are unable to understand the response in terms of the actor's frame of reference, intentions, motives, or desires in ways that fit the observers' theories about the wellsprings of human action.'[10] Torrey, of course, understands the talk; that is, he understands it from a clinical perspective – the talk is an instance of a clang association.

Rosenberg would characterize this interaction as an instance of role-taking failure – 'What makes the behavior insane is not so much the presence of distress or disability as the failure in role-taking.'[11] Rosenberg's comment, however, is problematic. It dichotomizes. Is insanity a social or a physical pathology? Does disability lead to the failure in role-taking or does the failure in role-taking lead to disability?

To dramatize the problem, consider what happens when, through the process of empathy, physicians do associate the action of an 'insane' member with what Rosenberg calls 'the wellsprings of human action.'[12] What happens when no 'radical rupture' exists between the afflicted and non-afflicted?

'I believe we will soon achieve world peace. But I'm still on the lamb.' Is it impossible to take the role of this writer diagnosed with schizophrenia? Is it impossible to hear this statement as meaningful? The speaker can be heard to be saying that, were world peace achieved, the lot of the speaker would remain poor and miserable. The speaker can be heard to be expressing a despair that stems from the suffering of schizophrenia, a despair that, as the speaker points out, is uninfluenced by utopian persuasions, whether they be medical or humanistic. Granting the confusion of the writing, the speaker can still be heard to be saying that he does not feel as if he is a part of the world. Given the brutish character of his affliction, he feels excluded from the advantages of the world.

This reading does not require either great depths of compassion or highly refined hermeneutical skills. An analysis of this writing which employed literary criticism or psychoanalysis might be more sophisticated in that the analysis might flesh out some esoteric irony. Perhaps the writer is asking: When will there be a cure for schizophrenia and when will I benefit from this cure? Perhaps the writer is asking: How mighty is medical science? What my reading shows is simply that, despite the confusion of the text, role-taking success is possible.[13]

To return to Rosenberg's account, is the 'insane' member no longer 'insane' when one associates the talk of an 'insane' member with 'the wellsprings of human action'? When no 'radical rupture' exists between the afflicted and non-afflicted, is there no longer the presence of disability?

Laing provides an idealistic answer to this question. He writes: 'The schizophrenic ceases to be schizophrenic when he meets someone with whom he feels understood. When this happens most of the bizarrerie which is taken as the "signs" of the "disease" simply evaporates.'[14] Consider the reality, though: If, to take the example that we have been considering, the writer felt that the despair that animates his writing had been genuinely understood, would the writer cease to be 'schizophrenic'? Would empathy cure the writer? The ability to take the role of someone with schizophrenia (which depends on a combination of numerous variables, such as imagination, energy, sensibilities, values, conditions, and experience) does not displace the fact that the person whose role we take suffers from a mental illness. Likewise, the ability of someone with schizophrenia to take the role of someone not afflicted with schizophrenia does not displace the fact that that person is afflicted with a mental illness.[15] In this light, consider a passage from Anne Deveson's *Tell Me I'm Here: One Family's Experience of Schizophrenia*:

To my surprise Jonathan hesitated, his head with that familiar tilt to one side. Then he said, 'Nuh.' He put his arms around me and cradled me as if I were the child, and he the parent. 'Don't cry, Anne.'[16]

Jonathan takes the role of his mother; that is, he shows empathy towards her suffering, and his mother is moved.

The argument being constructed here is atypical in that it does not dichotomize. The argument resists as well as supports Torrey's positivism. The argument supports as well as resists Laing's idealism. Unless one reasons as an idealist, to understand an afflicted member's talk as meaningful and intelligible does not displace the symptomatic nature of the member's talk, that is, the conditions from within which the speaker speaks and the actor lives. Likewise, unless one reasons as a positivist, to understand the member's talk as a symptom of pathology does not dictate that 'There is no logical association between "lamb" and "lam" except for their similar sound.' Laing's idealism is right – the writing is not mindless chatter. Torrey's positivism is right – the writing is an instance of a clang association.

Laing's idealism and Torrey's positivism are each required and each resisted in order to exemplify the perspective of analytic realism to which this study is committed. (Precedent for such an approach is set by Talcott Parsons.)[17] If role-taking success occurs between a physician and a patient, the reality of the affliction – that is, its pain and distress – does not disappear. What does disappear is the stigmatizing of the person with an affliction. When role-taking success occurs, what happens is that the afflicted person ceases to be judged 'schizophrenic.' 'Schizophrenic' is a prejudicial term that does not do justice to the humanity of the afflicted individual any more than does any other prejudicial term.[18]

An excellent example of this point is found in Torrey's reference to a Balzac short story. The story's narrator is the devoted wife of a man with schizophrenia. 'Perhaps nowhere,' Torrey says, 'is [the patience and understanding required for responding to a human being suffering from schizophrenia] better illustrated than by Balzac's heroine in "Louis Lambert."'[19] Torrey cites the following passage from the story:

'No doubt Louis appears to be "insane,"' she said, 'but he is not so, if the word insanity is applied only to those whose brain, from unknown causes, becomes vitiated, and who are, therefore, unable to give a reason for their acts. The equilibrium of my husband's mind is perfect. If he does not recognize you corporeally, do not think that he has not seen you. He is able to disengage his body and to see us under another form, I know not of what nature. When he speaks, he says marvelous things. Only, in fact often, he completes in speech an idea begun in the silence of his mind, or else he begins a proposition in words and finishes it mentally. To other men he must appear insane; to me, who lives in his thought, all his ideas are lucid. I follow the path of his mind; and though I cannot understand many of its turnings and digressions, I nevertheless reach the end with him.'[20]

Torrey qualifies his commendation of this text with the comment: 'Such dedication and understanding, unachievable except in fiction, is a worthy ideal.'[21] To develop a viable sociology of schizophrenia, it is, however, necessary to ask how this fictional example (which is worthy of imitation) can be rendered less ideal and more achievable. What sociological principle guides the wife's relation to her husband?

Role-taking success does not eradicate our understanding of another as mentally ill; Louis's wife neither glosses over nor denies the nature of her husband's affliction. Role-taking success, however, does eradicate the understanding of the afflicted member as a social leper and someone who is powerless. There is no causal correlation, but there is a sociological correlation between role-taking failure and the pathology of schizophrenia.

Although Rosenberg overlooks this point in his account of insanity as a social construction, he does point out a parallel qualification: 'There is in fact a large class of cases of role-taking failure that are *not* interpreted as insanity.'[22] For instance, if I understand a colleague's behaviour as weird, I indicate that I am unable to take the role of my colleague or, at best, do so only partially. I do not, however, necessarily judge my colleague (whose role I fail to take) to be insane.

The reason for the difference, Rosenberg says, is explained by attribution theory. In the one case, I attribute my failure to take the role of the other to myself (an internal attribution). In the other case, I attribute my failure to take the role of the other to the other (an external attribution). In the first case, no understanding of the other as insane is constructed. I simply lack the experience or knowledge to take the role of my colleague. In the second case, an understanding of the other as insane is constructed. My colleague is mentally ill and needs professional help.

Rosenberg's use of attribution theory does not, however, carry as much weight as it seems to. If I understand a colleague's behaviour as 'weird,' I may reason that I cannot take the role of the other because of the other as much as myself. I may reason that the basis for my failure is due both to the other (an external attribution) and to myself (an internal attribution). In other words, this distinction between external and internal is misleading. When is an external cause not also internal? When is an internal cause not also external? In social discourse, the two always go hand in hand.[23]

Sociology needs to stop asking how interactional issues such as role-taking failure ('this radical rupture in the role-taking process') determine psychosis and start asking how psychosis (as an incurable pathology) generates problematic but repairable interactional issues such as role-taking failure. The task for sociology is, not to assert a causal relation between role-taking failure and schizophrenia, but to explain the sociological foundation for the correlation between the two.

Egocentric Speech

The right question, then, is what is it about schizophrenia that leads to role-taking failure? Many answers can be given, but for our purposes, I will focus on one promoted by Rosenberg. Rosenberg says that there are two kinds of speech in social discourse – instrumental speech and expressive speech. 'Instrumental speech serves as a means to an end.' For instance, with instrumental speech I may 'wish to inform, to enlighten, to amuse, to convince, to frighten, to activate, to excite, to calm, to confuse, to mislead, to distract, to insult, or to produce any of an enormous number of general and specific effects on other people's minds.' My speech is a means to an end, the end being however I define my self-interest. 'Among adults,' Rosenberg asserts, 'most speech is instrumental.' For Rosenberg, the more developed the speaker, the more instrumental his or her speech. The less developed the speaker, the less instrumental his or her speech.[24]

By way of contrast, 'expressive speech (non–role-taking speech) ... is an end in itself. It is not intended to produce an impact on the mind of the listener but to verbalize the thoughts that cross the speaker's mind.' Expressive speech is just for itself, and it has no purpose outside of that. Children's language is an example of expressive speech – it seems asocial and solipsistic. For Rosenberg, the less developed the speaker, the more expressive his or her speech.[25]

Rosenberg inherits this distinction from Jean Piaget, but Rosenberg's presentation of the distinction distorts Piaget's actual argument. 'Expressive speech' is a term that resonates with what Piaget refers to as 'egocentric speech.' But the way in which Rosenberg formulates expressive speech makes it resonate more with what Piaget refers to as 'autism': 'Autistic thought ... is individualistic and obeys a set of special laws of its own.'[26]

Likewise, Rosenberg's notion of instrumental speech resonates with what Piaget refers to as 'directed thought.' For Piaget, 'autistic thought' is the opposite of 'directed thought'; for Rosenberg, expressive speech is the opposite of instrumental speech, speech that follows the logic of social intelligence.

Piaget's distinction between egocentric speech and social speech, however, is not as simple as Rosenberg would lead us to believe. The central argument in Piaget's work is that egocentric talk 'stands midway between autism in the strict sense of the word and socialized thought.'[27] Egocentric speech is intermediary; it is neither purely autistic nor fully socialized. This is what makes it so interesting. For Piaget, egocentric speech is qualitatively distinct from autistic thought. Egocentric speech is not unlike directed speech, which follows the logic of social intelligence.

Rosenberg, however, writes as if egocentric speech were autistic speech; his term 'expressive speech' thus reduces the significance of what egocentric speech is. Rosenberg collapses the dialectic that, according to Lev Vygotsky, is central to appreciating Piaget's studies of egocentric speech, and, in so doing, Rosenberg distorts Piaget's crucial points.

It is important to return to these primary materials from psychology from which Rosenberg develops his theory of insanity in order to critique Rosenberg's work and restore its capacity to explain the correlation between role-taking failure and schizophrenia. Rosenberg argues that the reason for role-taking failure is that the language of people with schizophrenia is expressive and not instrumental. Torrey, for example, is unable to take the role of the writer who says, 'I believe we will soon achieve world peace. But I'm still on the lamb,' because the writing is expressive rather than instrumental. The writing is child-like in that its central purpose is, not to communicate to another, but to express the thoughts that cross the mind of the writer. The text is an end in itself. Rosenberg reasons that, when language is expressive (that is, autistic and solipsistic) rather than instrumental (that is, spoken as a way to persuade others), 'normals' cannot be expected to take the role of people with schizophrenia.

To say that the language of people with schizophrenia is expressive, and to mean by 'expressive' autistic, is, however, to construct a caricature. When Rosenberg characterizes the language of people with schizophrenia as autistic, he provides a bogus rationalization for role-taking failure. He blames the victim. One way to resist Rosenberg's argument (and, as will be seen, it is not even the strongest way) is to restore the idea of expressive speech back to its original antecedent – namely, egocentric speech rather than autistic speech. This restoration counters Rosenberg's caricature. If we see the language of people with schizophrenia as egocentric, that is, intermediary between autistic and directed thought, rather than as autistic, our ability to hear the language of people with schizophrenia is changed. Our capacities for empathy are increased.

This argument is well supported by a recent documentary titled *A Place to Come Back To*, which examines the mission of the church and its response to the plight of people with mental illness.[28] One of the poignant moments in the documentary is when Mary Prothro, a church volunteer in Washington, DC, shares this experience:

Recently there's one man who ... really is not very attractive-looking. He has features that are ... not very good. His saliva comes out when he talks. But I was sitting at the table with him and another man said to me, 'Are you blessed?' And I said, 'Well, not in the Presbyterian Church. [laugh] That's sort of Catholic.' And this man ... said, 'She blessed.' And I looked at him. And he said, 'She blessed 'cause she sits at the table with me.'

How we conceive of people with schizophrenia determines how we interact with people with schizophrenia. If we see the behaviour of people with schizophrenia as autistic, that is, asocial, we relate one way. If we see the behaviour of people with schizophrenia as egocentric, and maybe even something stronger, we relate another way. In the interaction that Mary Prothro describes, she experienced a paradigm shift with respect to how she understood people with schizophrenia. This shift occurred as a result of this man showing empathy towards the awkwardness the Protestant volunteer felt when asked 'Are you blessed?' and taking the volunteer's role as a fellow Christian.

Rosenberg's sociological explanation of the language of people with schizophrenia regrettably reinforces society's prejudice towards people with schizophrenia. It is important, therefore, to critique his argument. There are two distortions here that need to be cleared up. One is that the language of people with schizophrenia represents a regression back to the autistic speech of a child. (Keep in mind that, for Piaget, egocentric speech is not autistic.) The second is that the limit of people with schizophrenia is defined by what the egocentric speech of a child is. The speech and reasoning of people with schizophrenia, while fragmented, problematic, and distorted, remains mature and cognitively developed. To cite Norman Cameron's well-chosen words: 'The disorganization seems to be really a process of disintegration rather than one of delamination.'[29]

If, when Rosenberg says that the language of people with schizophrenia is expressive, he means that the language of people with schizophrenia is egocentric (something intermediary between autistic and directed language), his theorizing would be less jarring. When one is experiencing pain, whether physical or psychological, an egocentric point of view is natural and understandable. Even this view, however, while sympathetic, is reductionistic.

Rosenberg's offence is that he privileges instrumental speech over expressive speech much as we saw Wolcott, in chapter 2, privilege semantic speech over poetic speech. The tension in this stratification is problematic, and the tension is confidently confronted in Vygotsky's review of Piaget's work on language development. Vygotsky's work asks us to question the value judgment in the distinction between instrumental and expressive speech. Why is the best speech that which is a means to an end? Why is the best speech that in which expressive speech (speech that is an end in itself) is absent? When instrumental speech dominates, what is it that is dominating, in so far as what dominates is speech whose intention is not to 'verbalize the thoughts that cross the speaker's mind'? What is instrumental speech's function in so far as its function is merely 'to produce an impact on the mind of the listener'? These questions challenge the distinction between instrumental speech and expressive speech, which Rosenberg uncritically employs to suggest a causal relation between role-taking failure and schizophrenia.

When Rosenberg says that the language of people with schizophrenia is primitive, he is focusing on what such language lacks – namely, an instrumental character, where for Rosenberg an instrumental character is what is essential to social speech.[30] Like many sociologists, Rosenberg reasons from a utilitarian perspective.[31] According to Vygotsky, however, the strength of Piaget's work is that 'Piaget concentrated on what the child *has* rather than on what the child lacks.' The key assumption of Piaget's study of children's language is that 'logical activity isn't all there is to intelligence.'[32] The offensive character in the distinction between instrumental and expressive language is that the distinction stipulates that logical activity is all there is to intelligence. Thus, in so far as people with schizophrenia fail to employ instrumental speech, they lack intelligence – they do not engage in socially determined logical activity.

If, by way of contrast, we embrace Piaget's notion that 'logical activity isn't all there is to intelligence,' the way in which we relate to and understand the language of people with schizophrenia changes. To say that the language of people with schizophrenia is non-logical is not to say that it is unintelligent.[33] Now we can start to ask more constructive questions. What is the intelligence of people with schizophrenia in so far as it is qualitatively distinct from socially determined logical activity? How is this intelligence expressed? How is it best understood?

Inner Speech

Vygotsky's writing encourages us to follow this path; his review of Piaget's work represents, first, a critique and, then, a development of Piaget's work. Vygotsky takes exception to Piaget's notion that, at a certain point in the child's development, egocentric speech disappears. Vygotsky confronts the implication that egocentric speech is inherently asocial. 'We have seen that egocentric speech is not suspended in a void but is directly related to the child's practical dealings with the real world.' Vygotsky accepts the distinction between egocentric and social speech, but he changes the terms of the distinction so as to undercut the suggestion that egocentric speech is asocial. Vygotsky argues that egocentric speech and directed speech are each social but that their functions are distinct. For Vygotsky (and here is the great irony), egocentric speech serves a more crucial function in human development than does directed speech. For Vygotsky, egocentric speech plays a transitional role in the transformation from vocal speech to inner speech. 'The true direction of the development of thinking is not from the individual to the socialized, but from the social to the individual.'[34] Egocentric speech is a precursor to inner speech, the foundation of human thought.

In Vygotsky's critique of Piaget, the stratification in the distinction between instrumental and expressive speech is inverted. Expressive speech *vis-à-vis* instrumental speech is formulated as showing a superior and more developed form of human thinking. In turn, instrumental speech becomes an inferior and less developed form of speech because instrumental speech does not develop into inner thought. To repeat: 'The true direction of the development of thinking is not from the individual to the socialized, but from the social to the individual.'

The purpose here is to explain the relation between role-taking failure and schizophrenia. Vygotsky repairs the flaws in Rosenberg's theorizing on this matter. If, when Rosenberg said that the language of people with schizophrenia represents a preponderance of expressive speech, he in fact meant that it represents a preponderance of inner speech, we would experience a significant inversion. We would keep the logic of Rosenberg's argument, but with a different attitude. A more adequate account of the language of people with schizophrenia is that it represents an externalization of inner speech. Vygotsky says that inner speech is 'to a large extent thinking in pure meanings. It is a dynamic, shifting, unstable thing, fluttering between word and thought, the two more or less stable, more or less firmly delineated components of verbal thought.'[35] The argument is more adequate both empirically and theoretically; it is also a more humane.

Let us return to the narrator in Balzac's short story, a text which Torrey highly commends:

Does it not often happen that while thinking of some trifling matter, we are drawn into serious thought by the gradual unfolding of ideas and recollections? Often, after speaking of some frivolous thing, the accidental point of departure for rapid meditation, a thinker forgets, or neglects to mention the abstract links which have led him to his conclusions, and takes up in speech only the last rings in the chain of reflections. Common minds to whom this quickness of mental vision is unknown, and who are ignorant of the inward travail of the soul, laugh at dreamers and call them madmen if they are given to such forgetfulness of connecting thoughts. Louis is always so; he wings his way through the spaces of thought with the agility of a swallow; yet I can follow him in all his circlings. That is the history of his so-called madness.[36]

The wife of the man with schizophrenia is clearly describing the language of her husband as an externalization of what Vygotsky means by 'inner speech'. Notice that the argument being constructed here is, in one sense, identical with the one from which we departed (role-taking failure); in another sense, it is different in that the caricature in the previous theory is jettisoned.

Consider again the questions that we asked earlier. That is, consider what happens when we repeat the questions, substituting Vygotsky's concept of inner speech for Rosenberg's notion of expressive speech.[37] Why is the best speech that in which inner speech is absent? When instrumental speech dominates, what is it that is dominating, in so far as it is the absence of inner speech? What is instrumental speech's purpose in so far as its purpose is distinct from the process of inner speech, that is, the process that reflects the speaker's mind and 'thinking in pure meaning'? The social message in the stratification that Rosenberg's theorizing creates is frightening.

Let me stress one straightforward point which fleshes out and exposes the problematic character of previous sociological studies of schizophrenia. To distinguish the sociological approach to insanity from the medical and psychiatric, Rosenberg states:

'Unlike the medical or psychiatric models, which anchor the problem of insanity in the individual, labeling theory and symbolic interactionism share a focus on the societal reaction to behavior.'[38] There is a problem with this distinction. If, like labelling theory, symbolic interaction examines, not so much the individual experiencing schizophrenia, but the societal reaction to the individual, how can symbolic interaction truly claim to be an interactional account? Why exclude the individual from the equation?[39] A sociological study which focuses on the societal reaction to the exclusion of the individual is ignoring something crucial. Why should sociology allow the individual to remain the exclusive domain of the medical and psychiatric professions? Can an adequate sociology of schizophrenia be developed if the afflicted individual (who is a social being) is excluded as part of the equation? Yes, the afflicted individual is subject to a medical and psychiatric account, but the individual, like all individuals, is also subject to a sociological analysis. Moreover, on certain points, the sociological analysis may be more tell-tale and more compelling than the medical or psychiatric.[40] Here is where a sociology of schizophrenia can intervene, and this intervention is needed. I pursue these issues in the next chapter in greater depth by examining the theorizing of postmodernism on schizophrenia as the glorification of 'inner speech.'[41] I now turn to the postmodern account of schizophrenia and the limit of the pariah.

4

THE INDIVIDUAL

Gilles Deleuze, Félix Guattari, and Jorge Luis Borges

But is it possible to understand everything? Is not the essence of mental illness, as opposed to normal behavior, precisely that it can be explained but that it resists all understanding?

— Michel Foucault[1]

Who is the individual who suffers the affliction known as schizophrenia? Does schizophrenia create an individual who is genuinely and radically different from other individuals? Is it even appropriate to speak of people with schizophrenia as having either social identities or human personalities?[2]

The person with schizophrenia is today's pariah, which is why postmodern thinkers like Michel Foucault, Gilles Deleuze, and Félix Guattari find the subject so appealing for their theorizing. The behaviour and language of people with schizophrenia seem to stand beyond the pale of rationality, not unlike the very theorizing of postmodernism itself. In postmodern writing, people with schizophrenia are exemplars of the ideal relation between the individual and society; people with schizophrenia are heuristic tools for postmodern pedagogy.[3] The purpose of this chapter is to explicate the postmodern understanding of schizophrenia and to address how postmodernism develops a sociology of schizophrenia even as postmodernism itself disdains such a project.

Chagrin

Harry Stack Sullivan stands as a precursor to the postmodern view of schizophrenia:[4]

I diagnose schizophrenia by certain types of disturbance of speech unaccompanied by chagrin, but I have yet to see a schizophrenic early in his illness who has not been chagrined by hearing himself say certain things to me which he recognized afterwards as incommunicative.[5]

Chagrin is when self's 'me' is aware of the contradictory behaviour and attitude of self's 'I.' Chagrin occurs with the recognition of a significant discordance between the two parts of self known as the 'me' and the 'I.' For example, chagrin may be exemplified through a blush; a blush is more than blood rushing to the face. It is a social phenomenon in that it displays self through a somatic appearance. It signifies self's recognition of a significant discordance between the parts of the self that Mead formulates as the 'me' ('the organized set of attitudes of others which one himself assumes') and the 'I' ('something that is never entirely calculable').[6] The blush is an icon of self's recognition of self.

With respect to self's 'me,' Mead writes: 'The "me" is the organized set of attitudes of others which one himself assumes. The attitudes of the others constitute the organized "me".'[7] With respect to self's 'I,' Mead writes: 'That action of "I" is something the nature of which we cannot tell in advance'; 'the "I" gives the sense of freedom, of initiative'; and 'the "I" is something that is never entirely calculable.'[8]

With respect to the interrelation between the 'I' and the 'me,' Mead writes: 'Taken together they constitute a personality as it appears in social experience. The self is essentially a social process going on with these two distinguishable phases. If it [self] did not have these two phases there could not be conscious responsibility, and there would be nothing novel in experience.'[9] An actor's blush in a social interaction signifies a discordance between self's 'me' and self's 'I' and the possible reintegration of these two parts of the self.

Sullivan says that schizophrenia is observed in 'certain types of disturbance of speech unaccompanied by chagrin.' 'Unaccompanied by chagrin' is the operative phrase here. Sullivan indicates that schizophrenia is evident when self's 'me' is absent or, to put it another way, when self's 'I' is all that appears to be present. We observe schizophrenia when an actor's 'I' rather than an actor's 'me' governs behaviour. This understanding of schizophrenia as a human phenomenon dominates psychology, as Louis A. Sass indicates when he critiques psychological texts: 'Schizophrenics are idiosyncratic, unique, inappropriate or bizarre ... any further elaboration is impossible.'[10] In other words, 'schizophrenics' are all 'I' and no 'me.' Schizophrenia is the waning of self-consciousness; when schizophrenia is florid, self-consciousness is non-existent.

This notion of schizophrenia dominates the social sciences. Laing makes use of Mead's distinction when he writes:

There is still an 'I' that cannot find a 'me.' An 'I' has not ceased to exist, but it is without substance, it is disembodied, it lacks the quality of realness, and it has no identity, it has no 'me' to go with it. It may seem a contradiction in terms to say that the 'I' lacks identity but this seems to be so. The schizophrenic either does not know who or what he is or he has become something or someone other than himself. At any rate, without such a last shred or scrap of a self, an 'I' therapy of any kind would be impossible.[11]

In Laing's theorizing, people with schizophrenia are divided in two senses: their selves are divided from their bodies, and their selves' 'I' are divided from their selves' 'me.' According to Laing, schizophrenia is observed in social discourse when a self's 'I' cannot find its 'me,' when a self's 'I' escapes capture by 'me.'

Anti-Oedipus: Capitalism and Schizophrenia

Does this notion represent an adequate understanding of what schizophrenia is as a human experience? Postmodern theorists answer with a resounding 'yes' and extend the notion which pervades Sullivan and Laing's work. For Sullivan and Laing, however, the notion of an 'I' detached from and unrelated to a 'me' is unhealthy. It represents a pathology, one which Sullivan and Laing, as physicians, seek to cure. By way of contrast, postmodern theorists view the notion of an 'I' detached from and unrelated to a 'me' as positive. It represents an escape from pathology. Society's pathology is exemplified in the oppressive and controlling relation 'me' has within the individual.[12]

Consider the following comment by Deleuze and Guattari: 'For the schizo is the one who escapes all Oedipal, familial, and persological references – I'll no longer say me, I'll no longer say daddy–mommy – and he keeps his word.'[13] The 'schizo' never 'arouses in himself the attitudes of others.' The schizo neither exemplifies nor sustains a 'me.'

In *Anti-Oedipus*, Deleuze and Guattari affirm the abondonment of 'me,' by 'I.' They insist that 'I' is absolute and 'me' is not so much secondary as irrelevant and insignificant. Deleuze and Guattari do not say that 'I' dominates 'me' (that would be the work of 'me') but that 'I' destroys 'me.' Their anarchistic humanism is that 'I' destroys 'me' for the purpose of restoring the human species back to its natural, individualistic, and authentic state.[14] For postmodern theorists, people with schizophrenia are marching in the vanguard.

Deleuze and Guattari articulate and formulate their view of schizophrenia *vis-à-vis* Laing's clinical view, and it is helpful to consider how Deleuze and Guattari distinguish their perspective from Laing's. Initially, Deleuze and Guattari praise Laing's work; they write: 'R.D. Laing is entirely right in defining the schizophrenic process a voyage of initiation, a transcendental experience of the loss of the Ego.'[15] With Laing, Deleuze and Guattari see schizophrenia as 'a transcendental experience of the loss of the Ego.'

Deleuze and Guattari, however, admonish Laing's understanding of schizophrenia. They critique Laing for not going far enough, for not appreciating the true implications of what they call 'the schizophrenic process':

At the very moment [Laing] breaks with psychiatric practice, undertakes assigning a veritable social genesis to psychosis, and calls for a continuation of the 'voyage' as a process and for a dissolution of the 'normal ego,' he falls back into the worst familialist, personological, and egoic postulates, so that the remedies invoked are no more than a 'sincere corroboration among parents,' a 'recognition of the real persons,' a discovery of the true ego or self as in Martin Buber.[16]

As theorists, Deleuze and Guattari see themselves as superior to Laing. What do they know that Laing does not? Where Laing goes wrong is with the assumption that the 'I' seeks an authentic 'me.' Deleuze and Guattari knock Laing for retaining the notion that there is something good and wholesome towards which self, by its nature, strives. Deleuze and Guattari disdain Laing's unwillingness to let go of what, for postmodernism, is a neurotic ideology – namely, the notion that the self can be both free and integrated. However unconventional Laing may be for mainstream psychologists, he is too straight for Deleuze and Guattari. Laing romantically believes in the possibility of 'a discovery of the true ego or self as in Martin Buber,' a principle that Deleuze and Guattari hold in contempt.[17]

For Deleuze and Guattari, the positive feature of schizophrenia as a human experience is that it discloses in all truth that the 'I' has no need 'to find a "me".'[18] Let it not be said that the theorizing of postmodernism is without conviction, without a commitment to what is irrefutable and necessary, without a notion of what is real. 'It is certain,' Deleuze and Guattari assert, 'that neither men nor women are clearly defined personalities, but rather vibrations, flows, schizzes, and "knots".'[19] For Deleuze and Guattari, the schizophrenic process is an emancipatory one because in the schizophrenic process the influence of 'me' is no longer significant.

The postmodern position violates what, for Mead, is a fundamental truth of human nature.[20] 'The "me" and the "I" lie in the process of thinking ... These two, as they appear in our experience, constitute the personality.'[21] From Mead's perspective, as long as the 'I' remains unrelated to and detached from 'me,' a person neither forms nor sustains a self. A person cannot think. A person has no personality.

Jorge Luis Borges

For the sake of conversation which produces constructive analysis, let us develop a compelling example of postmodernism's notion of the schizophrenic process. Let us consider the postmodern understanding of schizophrenia from the strongest vantage point possible. Jorge Luis Borges wrote an essay titled 'Borges and I'; the essay narrates poignantly the dialectic between 'I' and 'me' as what self is.[22] Among postmodern intellectuals, Borges is a popular author, and this essay would no doubt be praised as a non-clinical example of what is meant by the schizophrenic process.

The essay begins: 'It's the other one, it's Borges, that things happen to.' Whose voice is speaking here and who is 'the other one' to whom the voice refers? The voice is self's 'I'; 'the other one' is self's 'me,' 'Borges.' 'I like hourglasses, maps, eighteenth-century typography, the taste of coffee, and Stevenson's prose. The other one shares these preferences with me, but in a vain way that converts them into attributes of an actor.' The tastes and pleasures of 'I' cannot themselves be conceptualized or cataloged. Those tastes and pleasures are random, conditional. Reason does not govern the listing of 'I.' Borges, 'the other one,' however, 'converts them into attributes of an actor.' 'Me' seizes the tastes and pleasures of 'I' such that they are no longer attributes of 'I' but attributes of an actor with an identity.[23]

The essay's voice laments being unable to live independently of 'me.' It laments its lack of freedom from 'me.' It laments the inevitable way in which 'the other one' co-opts its nature and destroys its original state. 'But I must live on in Borges, not in myself – if indeed I am anyone – though I recognize myself less in his books than in many others, or than in the laborious strumming of a guitar.' The essay's voice shows no need for identity, no need to be an actor with personality. The essay's voice compares itself to 'the laborious strumming of a guitar.' Ironically, the voice recognizes itself more in books written by others than in those written by Borges.[24]

The dialectic here is that, while 'I' laments its subjection to 'me,'

'I' grounds the possibility of self-consciousness. 'Me' detached from and unrelated to an 'I' is not self-consciousness; it is what is known in the literature as an authoritarian personality. 'I' allows for and generates the conversation of self that is called reflexiveness. 'Years ago I tried to free myself from him and I passed from lower-middle-class myths to playing games with time and infinity, but those games are Borges's now, and I will have to conceive something else.'[25]

Postmodern theorists would point to Borges's essay as a model of the schizophrenic process. The essay shows 'I' as absolute and the 'me' as parasitic, and yet, at the same time, the 'I' is nothing and the 'me' is everything. Here is the great epistemology, the ineffable paradox, to which postmodern philosophers are so committed.[26]

What postmodernism refuses to acknowledge is the synthesis of 'I' and 'me' as the work and product of reflexiveness. What it does not recognize is the dialectical relation between 'I' and 'me' as the grounds for identity and self development. Borges's essay concludes: 'I do not know which of us two is writing this page.' Is this concluding line tragic or comic? This concluding line is tragic if 'me' has co-opted once again the last thread of the distinctiveness of 'I.' It is comic if 'I,' in its final speaking, has retained a thread of existence that 'me,' Borges, can neither cut nor tie. The beauty of this concluding line is that it is both.

Does postmodernism portray people with schizophrenia as they are or as postmodernism would have them be? Does postmodernism co-opt the experience of schizophrenia according to its own agenda? What does the postmodern understanding have to do with the experience of schizophrenia?[27] I recommend reserve towards the postmodern perspective because it seems to be more of an intellectual projection, albeit clever and dialectical, than a humane and sympathetic response to the experience of schizophrenia.[28]

It is clear that what Mead speaks of as self's 'me' – taking on the attitudes of others and society towards self, and thus constituting a self – is present in the language and behaviour of people with schizophrenia. Before the onslaught of this illness, the person had a self, a self mediated by a dynamic relation between 'me' and 'I.'

There is no reason to think that, upon incurring the affliction, the individual suddenly lacks a self. People suffering from schizophrenia experience pride and shame, honour and guilt (the characteristics of self's 'me') to the same degree and with the same quality as someone not suffering from schizophrenia.

People with schizophrenia, for instance, express shame that they are afflicted with schizophrenia, and society does little to discourage this shame. They also express astute judgments about themselves, others, and their social world. It is common for people with schizophrenia to express what Mead speaks of as 'the generalized other' and to articulate statements with respect to who they are as human beings and their values as members of society. There are many examples of this point in the 'First Person Accounts' on the last page of each issue of *Schizophrenia Bulletin* published by the National Institute for Mental Health. (The inclusion of these accounts is enlightened and humane, but the National Institute of Mental Health does not seem to view them as material for research.)

Love

Schizophrenia is a disease that leaves the self distraught but does not change or alter the basic structure of self. The self is too strong to be overpowered by this affliction. Despite the rhetorical arguments of postmodern intellectuals, schizophrenia does not create an individual who is genuinely and radically different from other individuals. Antonin Artaud, for instance, is not different from anybody else; he is 'normal' in that he is self-conscious. His reflexiveness and intellectualizing exemplify, not a loss, but a retention of self.[29]

While reserve towards the postmodern perspective is recommended, it is important to retain one crucial feature of the postmodern perspective. Unlike most approaches in the social sciences, the postmodern perspective insists upon recognizing people with schizophrenia as compelling subjects by recognizing the agency of people with schizophrenia, which is exactly what other approaches in the social sciences fail to do.

Postmodern theorists, however, would object to the use of the term 'agency' to describe their position because 'agency' is the last thing that they see people with schizophrenia possessing. Indeed, it is the very thing that they see people with schizophrenia break through.[30] It is easy, however, to reconcile the tension in this reading of postmodernism and its understanding of schizophrenia. The problem with the postmodern understanding of schizophrenia is that agency is all that the postmodern perspective recognizes. It treats agency as absolute, and, when absolute, agency has neither limit nor reality.

Consider the following comment by Deleuze and Guattari: 'Schizophrenia is like love: there is no specifically schizophrenic phenomenon or entity.'[31] What is it to assert that schizophrenia is like love? The comment strikes anyone who is familiar with people afflicted with schizophrenia as cruel and thoughtless. There is nothing lovable about schizophrenia in and of itself, although people with schizophrenia are certainly lovable human beings.

What is it then for Deleuze and Guattari to say that schizophrenia is like love? When in love, agency is all that seems to matter. When in love, other matters such as conditions, circumstances, family, space, time, values, and structure are insignificant. When one is in love, agency becomes omnipotent. Think of Romeo and Juliet; not even death was a significant limit for their love, although it was a significant limit for them. Love leads to tragedy because, as agency becomes absolute, it loses power, and therefore significance. If we understand the limit of love as the limit of agency as it becomes absolute, the comments by Deleuze and Guattari make perfect sense. Consider their slogan – 'We would like to speak in the name of absolute incompetence.'[32] In some ways, postmodernism resembles a secular Christianity; consider the following biblical passages as postmodern lessons for everyday life – 'God chose what is low and despised in the world, even things that are not, to bring to nothing things that are' (1 Corinthians 1: 28) or 'For the foolishness of God is wiser than men, and the weakness of God is stronger than men' (1 Corinthians 1: 25).

Why are postmodern theorists enamoured with schizophrenia? They are fixated on agency, and, when it comes to understanding action, they cannot tolerate the presence of any variables other than agency – for instance, other actors, conditions, social structure, competing means, compelling ends, or norms. They love agency to the exclusion of all other features of social action. Postmodern theorists are right – there is no action without agency. They are also wrong – there is no action when agency is all that is significant.

Lev Vygotsky's comments on inner speech are helpful at this point because they provide an image of what agency looks like when seen as something absolute, of what it looks like independent of anything else. Agency is aligned with inner speech; inner speech is the grounds for agency, which is what makes agency something that cannot be quantified by social science.[33] Vygotsky writes:

Inner speech is to a large extent thinking in pure meanings. It is a dynamic, shifting, unstable thing, fluttering between word and thought, the two more or less stable, more or less firmly delineated components of verbal thought.[34]

Postmodern theorists are enamoured with schizophrenia because, as a human phenomenon, schizophrenia looks like inner speech before being transformed and so distorted into articulate, that is, social, speech. The language and behaviour of people with schizophrenia resemble thought before it is made concretely intelligible and meaningful. To put it another way, the language of people with schizophrenia is full of sense (it is suggestive, sensitive), but completely lacking in meaning (it lacks sociability, communicativeness).

Postmodern theorists are enamoured with schizophrenia because schizophrenia seems to provide a direct view of inner speech. For postmodern theorists, it provides an icon of what thought is before it is rendered intelligible in social discourse. Schizophrenia looks like pure thought before it is disfigured by language.

This discussion of the postmodern understanding of schizophrenia leads to a practical question for those who treat and live with people with schizophrenia. Does reflexiveness – as a dynamic relation between thought and word – lead to self-development or does it lead to 'loss of self'? Are the gains garnered from reflexiveness for someone with schizophrenia any different from those garnered by someone without schizophrenia? For instance, is psychotherapy, as, let us say, a safe site which nurtures and encourages reflexiveness, an appropriate or inappropriate treatment for people with schizophrenia?

Torrey strongly promotes one side of the argument:

To do insight-oriented psychotherapy on persons with schizophrenia is analogous to directing a flood into a town already ravaged by a tornado or, to use another comparison from a recent review entitled 'The Adverse Effects of Intensive Treatment of Chronic Schizophrenia,' insight-oriented psychotherapies are 'analogous to pouring boiling oil into wounds because they ignore the chronic schizophrenic's particular vulnerability to overstimulating relationships, intense negative affects, and pressures for rapid change.'[35]

While stated in a vituperate manner, Torrey's arguments make sense, especially in light of our preceding discussion. Laing's psychoanalytic treatment did more harm than good for his patients because he focused only on the labour of agency – namely, reflexiveness – and ignored conditions – namely, the diseased body. Laing believed that reflexiveness – as a method of psychoanalysis, could in and of itself cure schizophrenia.

Susan Sheehan softly promotes the other side of the argument. Insight-oriented psychotherapy helped her subject Sylvia, that is, helped Sylvia, not with her schizophrenia, but with her self-understanding as a young adult and a human being. Sheehan cites a clinical report from an insight-oriented psychotherapist named Francine Baden who treated Sylvia:

Despite the pathology, it is felt that this youngster has real strengths, and is fighting to integrate herself, and to be well and happy, and to separate herself from her family (although there is enormous conflict, anxiety and guilt about it). She is unusually bright, talented, sensitive, and has rich potentialities. It is felt that a very warm, strong and positive relationship has been established with the therapist.[36]

Baden continues:

Considering the extensive pathology of this family, particularly the fantastic pressure of the mother, her profound rejection and hostility of Sylvia, her clutching demandingness and hysterical reactions, it speaks for Sylvia's strengths that she is so desperately trying to pull away.[37]

If insight-oriented psychotherapy strengthens a person by increasing self-awareness, ought the person with schizophrenia to be excluded from such strengthening?

5

PUNS

Kenneth Burke and M.M. Bakhtin

Through this victory, laughter clarified man's consciousness and gave him a new outlook on life.

– M.M. Bakhtin[1]

As I walk past a mainstream church in a small midwestern town on a hot summer day, I read the following statement: 'Come, Praise the Summer, Son.' As I continue, I walk past a jeweller's display window in which I read: 'A carat or more won't spoil her diet.' Inside the window are three orange, cloth carrots with green tops, one of which is wearing a diamond ring.

We encounter puns all the time in everyday life. Elaine Chaika writes: 'In recent years, American advertising has been characterized by a fit of punning.'[2] We also encounter puns, or what seem to be puns, in schizophrenic language. The following example of illogical thinking is cited in a diagnostic manual of the American Psychiatric Association. A clinician asks a patient to define *parents*, and the patient responds:

Parents are the people that raise you. Anything that raises you can be a parent. Parents can be anything, material, vegetable, or mineral, that has taught you something. Parents would be the world of things that are alive, that are there. Rocks, a person can look at a rock and learn something from it, so that would be a parent.[3]

In this chapter, we ask if humour and pathology are mutually exclusive. Is it inappropriate to laugh at this example of 'illogical thinking' from a psychotic patient? Is the humour that we might experience from this talk completely unrelated to the speaker and the talk itself?

Here are the questions that need to be addressed: What is a pun? What is the significance of a pun sociologically? Is there a difference between the punning of people with schizophrenia and that of people not afflicted with schizophrenia? If a difference exists, how can the difference be formulated and understood? If the argument can be made that those with schizophrenia do in fact pun, what is the significance of this action?

Perspective by Incongruity

Kenneth Burke again provides the materials with which to address these matters. He provides a working concept of what the pun is in social discourse:

Perspective by incongruity, or 'planned incongruity,' is a methodology of the pun ... Literally, a pun links by tonal association words hitherto unlinked ... It is 'impious' as regards our linguistic categories established by custom.[4]

To go back to my initial examples, the statement on the church sign, 'Come Praise the Summer, Son,' is a pun in that it links through tonal association words hitherto unlinked – 'sun' and 'Son.' The statement is a pun, given the uncustomary linkage of two semantically dissimilar words. Likewise, 'A carat or more won't spoil her diet' links two tonally similar words, 'carat' and 'carrot,' with two unrelated contexts, a woman's finger and a carrot. The carrot wearing a diamond ring visualizes the pun.

What, though, about the example of 'illogical thinking'? The patient defines parents as 'people that raise you.' An acceptable answer. The patient then does a parody of the definition: The patient suggests different signifiers, 'material, vegetable, or mineral,' which could substitute for what the signifier *parents* signifies. At the end of the talk, 'rock' becomes a substitute for what the signifier *parents* signifies. While unexpected, 'rock' represents a logical progression in that it is an antonym for the preceding reference – 'the world of things that are alive.' The pun, in so far as there is one, is to think of 'rocks' as a signifier of what parents are. There is a pun here in so far as 'rock' becomes a sign instead of another arbitrary signifier.[5] Many could find humour in the idea of a rock as a sign for 'parents' – it affirms an adolescent's mythology of what parents are.

Of course, not every sign is a pun. In this case, 'rock' is a sign *qua* pun in so far as it, in Burke's words, is '"impious" as regards our linguistic categories established by custom.'

In *Understanding Psychotic Speech: Beyond Freud and Chomsky,* Chaika concludes with a series of pressing questions which insist upon a sociological examination of the subject:

If the schizophrenic's meaning can be so very far removed from normals, how does anyone know what the schizophrenic means? At what point in a patient's illness does one suspend the normal rules of decoding and substitute the schizophrenic ones? At what point in remission does one abandon the schizophrenic interpretations and go back to the ones shared by other speakers? Or is the schizophrenic's speech always governed by the rules of schizophrenia? If so, should these rules be applied retroactively, say, perhaps, to five years before the visible onset of illness? Or does one start interpreting differently at the precise moment when schizophrenic illness is diagnosed?[6]

These questions are as much sociological as they are clinical or linguistic.[7] The possible answers to these questions have serious implications for people with schizophrenia. What would it mean, for example, upon the onset of schizophrenia, to have one's talk retroactively interpreted according to schizophrenic rather than normal rules of decoding?[8] What are these schizophrenic rules of decoding? Can people who are not afflicted with schizophrenia construct these 'schizophrenic rules' *vis-à-vis* 'normal rules'? Is the nature of these schizophrenic rules simply that they rule out the speaker as a meaningful participant in a dialogic relation?[9]

As indicated, our interest in puns is not in their production as a linguistic achievement, which linguists call 'paronomasia,' but in their meaningfulness in social discourse, both for those afflicted and for those not.[10] Paul Thibault writes:

Paronomasia is one form of rhetorical code switching which requires both addresser and addressee to make a series of careful ontological decisions. Paronomasia is basically a rhetorical figure of speech. The rules of rhetoric allow for the substitution of a word and corresponding concept with other words and concepts.[11]

Following this lead, what is the rhetorical code that allows for a switching or substitution of a word for its corresponding concept? What is the rhetorical code that allows for an apparent arbitrary signifier to become a human sign? Whence comes this understanding that permits both the addresser and the addressee to make this switching? What would it mean for this switching to be short-circuited, as appears to be the case in interactions with people with schizophrenia?

Let us look at a 'normal' example. When I read the sign in the church yard, 'Come, Praise the Summer, Son,' I make the switching required to appreciate the playfulness of the statement. When I read 'A carat or more won't spoil her diet,' I make the substitution required given the code of this particular text. When, however, we hear 'Rocks, a person can look at a rock and learn something from it, so that would be a parent,' why is the switching that is required for a successful pun less likely to occur? Why does the decoding that facilitates punning break down? Is there another code, a schizophrenic code, that overrides the normal code such that we are unable to hear the clinical example as punning? That is, what are the ontological decisions that are made such that the clinical example is a failed pun and the church sign and jeweller's display window successful puns?

If there are rules of decoding that provide for the switching in one case and not the other, what are these metarules for when and when not to employ normal rules of decoding? Is it possible to formulate these metarules such that, in the case of illogical thinking, they might be overridden so as to treat illogical thinking as an instance of punning? Would such a reading of illogical thinking constitute a 'stretch'? What would allow for this 'stretching,' and how could we establish the metarule that permits the stretching required to hear what a clinician calls 'illogical thinking' as an instance of punning?

Using the notion of 'perspective by incongruity,' Burke formulates the significance of puns:

The metaphorical extension of perspective by incongruity involves casuistic stretching, since it interprets new situations by removing words from their 'constitutional' setting. It is not 'demoralizing,' however, since it is done by the 'transcendence' of a new start. It is not negative smuggling, but positive cards-face-up-on-the-table. It is designed to 'remoralize' by accurately naming the situation already demoralized by inaccuracy.[12]

Burke formulates the pun as an act. The interesting character of a pun is that its reasoning, based on an unlikely linkage of two hitherto unconnected words, is misleading – casuistic. The reasoning is sophistical. Casuistic is a loaded term; it carries a lot of weight for Burke's formulation of what a pun is. Let us consider some examples.

Consider the church sign 'Come, Praise the Summer, Son.' The association of 'Son' and 'sun' creates an 'impious' connection. The sign calls people to church. What is it that calls people to church? The Son of God or the sun? In linking these two tonally similar words, the pun suggests an interchangeability, and the interchangeability transgresses conventional Christian sensibility. Does the sun, a pagan image, call Christians to worship or does the Son of God, Jesus? Upon reflection, the sign might offend a Christian but amuse a rhetorician. The sign's reasoning is casuistic.

Is the logic and construction of the pun so different from what clinicians call 'illogical thinking,' 'thinking that contains obvious internal contradictions or in which conclusions are reached that are clearly erroneous, given the initial premises'? What is the difference between puns in 'normal' talk and puns in 'schizophrenic' talk? Can we formulate a difference and, at the same time, preserve a similarity?

This critical reading of 'Come, Praise the Summer, Son' contrasts with Burke's more generous understanding of the significance of pun in social discourse. The minister who made the sign did not see what he or she was doing as heresy. Nor did he or she see it as demoralizing for Christian practice. The minister's purpose was positive, not demoralizing. The context in which the statement is made is a hot summer. The pun interprets the new situation, the midwestern summer, by removing a word from its 'constitutional' setting and placing it in a contrasting and unusual setting. The pun achieves a 'transcendence,' which, symbolically, represents a new start. From the minister's point of view, the sign is pious. 'It is designed to "remoralize" by accurately naming the situation already demoralized by inaccuracy.' Hot summer days, however unpleasant, are God's creation, and Christians need to be 'remoralized' on this point.[13]

Why analyse the dialogic character of puns in 'normal' discourse? Because it is important for an adequate appreciation of puns or what appear to be puns in schizophrenic discourse. What we are doing is taking puns in normal talk and showing how they are not unlike schizophrenic language.[14] The point here is that what it means to be normal, to use speech that follows normal rules of decoding, needs to questioned and appraised. We must question what it means to be normal so as to encompass rather than exclude speakers with schizophrenia.[15]

Consider the pun in the jeweller's window, 'A carat or more won't spoil her diet.' Beneath the sign are three orange cloth carrots with green tops; one of the carrots is wearing a diamond ring.[16] The pun represents a 'planned incongruity.' 'It is "impious" as regards our linguistic categories established by custom.' Feeding her a carrot becomes interchangeable with buying her a diamond ring. A carrot or more becomes analogous with a carat or more. The insignificant cost of a few more carrots becomes equivalent with the considerable cost of a diamond with a few more carats. The reasoning of the pun is casuistic; it stretches reality; it glosses truth. If this statement were spoken by someone with schizophrenia, would a psychologist characterize the pun as 'glossomania' – 'a chaining in which shared meanings of words progress linearly ... from one phrase to another, getting progressively further and further away from whatever meaning was apparently intended'?[17]

The element of misogyny in this pun should not be overlooked. 'A carat or more won't spoil her diet' equates the woman's desire for jewellery with an animal's appetite for food – both seem insatiable. This correspondence is reinforced (by inversion) with the word 'spoil.' Spoil operates as an antonym as well as a *double entendre*. On the one hand, by buying her a larger diamond ring, the buyer spoils her with affection. On the other hand, by feeding her a carrot, the buyer won't spoil her diet. To repeat the paradox, on the one hand, the woman's appetite for food is something that she controls for the sake of her figure. On the other hand, her desire for jewellery is something she cannot control. Wouldn't it be nice to spoil, that is, kill, her appetites with this large diamond ring? Hostility and love, aggression and compassion, come together and become interchangeable.[18] Buying her a diamond ring is defined as manliness, and manliness is represented through a concealed hatred towards women. Such are the ontological decisions which allow for the appreciation of this pun and which ensure that the addresser and the addressee make the necessary switches to appreciate the pun. Note the *double entendre*, 'spoil,' (which is what he does when he buys her the diamond ring) also means 'putrefy.'

As before, this critical reading of the pun serves as a background to Burke's more generous reading of the significance of puns in social discourse. The jeweller who created this pun was not conscious of the interpretations offered above, which is not to say that the jeweller does not reason. From the jeweller's perspective, the purpose of the pun is to attract potential customers. Who wants to spend a lot of money for a diamond ring? The pun reframes what it means to buy a diamond in order to alleviate the pain of the cost. When cast as something as natural and healthy as eating carrots, purchasing the diamond ring becomes less painful. Is the casuistic logic of the pun, the sophistical reasoning of the pun, not crazy?

It should be noted that some oppose the argument being developed here. Chaika writes:

Unusual word choices abound in witticisms, good prose, and artistic language, but these are quite different from schizophrenic unusual word choices. Witticisms, good prose, and artistic language in some way elucidate a message in a memorable or aesthetic manner. In contrast, schizophrenic 'unusual' word choices rarely have any such relevance.[19]

According to Chaika, schizophrenic discourse is dysfunctional language:

The problem is that the productions are not subordinated to form or to a coherent meaning. They are not controlled, and control is the essence of art and of ordinary communication.[20]

Schizophrenic language is language where, to use Mead's terms, 'me' is completely absent or inoperative. There is no control, and therefore language is asocial. It lacks what it needs to be language: a 'me.' Notice how Chaika embraces the same conception of people with schizophrenia as do the postmodern theorists.[21]

There are two ways to confront this position.[22] One is to point out, as postmodern theorists do, the inflated significance of control in Chaika's writing. Are normal speakers in as much control as we typically think they are? For instance, do the author of the church sign and the designer of the jeweller's display window fully reflect on what they are saying? Are they in full control of the meaningfulness of their language? Is everything that they say everything that they wanted to say? Is something said that is not intended, as in the case of the *faux pas*? Vygotsky helps us to make this point when he writes:

Thought and word are not cut from one pattern. In a sense, there are more differences than likenesses between them. The structure of speech does not simply mirror the structure of thought; that is why words cannot be put on by thought like a ready-made garment. Thought undergoes many changes as it turns into speech. It does not merely find expression in speech; it finds its reality and form.[23]

A second way to confront Chaika's position is to stress that in schizophrenic language there is not so much an absence of self's 'me' as an atypical expression of self's 'me.' 'Me' is still operative but in a way that takes into account and struggles with the schizophrenia. 'Me' is still active, if only in the sense that self takes the point of view of what it is to be a human being and what it is for a human being to be afflicted with schizophrenia. While psychotic speech may be unintelligible as what Piaget calls 'directed speech', it is full of meaning when recognized as an inverted reflection of inner speech.[24] Psychotic speech is human speech rather than animal communication because its source, like all human speech, is not speech, but thought.

The Beauty of the Grotesque

It is time to introduce and analyse examples of puns in schizophrenic discourse. Do people with schizophrenia pun? How is the punning of people with schizophrenia different? If a difference exists, how is the difference to be formulated and understood? If people with schizophrenia do pun, what is the significance of this action?

Charlie Chaplin and Buster Keaton demonstrate that puns can be made through behaviour as much as through language. Given this point, consider the following anecdote from Gregory Bateson's study 'Toward a Theory of Schizophrenia':

On a ward with a dedicated and 'benevolent' physician in charge, there was a sign on the physician's door which said 'Doctor's Office. Please Knock.' The doctor was driven to distraction and finally capitulation by the obedient patient who carefully knocked every time he passed the door.'[25]

Let us then consider the example of 'the obedient patient who carefully knocks every time he passed the door.'[26] If we saw

Charlie Chaplin or Buster Keaton perform this routine on screen, we would laugh. However, when reported in a clinical fashion as it is by Bateson, the behaviour looks pathetic, incompetent.[27]

Let us, though, assume that the patient is oriented: 'Social action ... may be oriented to the past, present, or expected future behavior of others.'[28] Let us assume that the patient comprehends the sign on the door – 'Doctor's Office. Please Knock.' Let us assume that the patient hears the sentence as an imperative, a command applicable in every instance.[29]

To construct the intelligibility of this behaviour, it helps to draw upon M.M. Bakhtin's formulation of the grotesque.

The grotesque liberates man from all the forms of inhuman necessity that direct the prevailing concept of the world ... Necessity, in every concept which prevails at any time, is always one-piece, serious, unconditional, and indisputable.[30]

The doctor's office represents the prevailing order of the mental hospital for the patient. The weight of this prevailing order is one of necessity. As a prevailing order, it is 'one-piece, serious, unconditional, and indisputable.' The obedient patient seems to be doing a parody of this prevailing order that governs his life-world. The patient is doing a caricature of the order under which he lives. By treating the sign on the doctor's door seriously, that is, too seriously, the patient reveals how unserious and insignificant the sign really is. To use Barthes's terms, the patient transforms the 'sign' of the sign into a mere 'signifier.' In doing this, the patient transforms the sign into something that is no more or less absurd than he is as someone with schizophrenia. The patient shares his madness by exposing the 'illogical thinking' of this sign on the door. As Burke would say, the behaviour is 'designed to "remoralize" by accurately naming the situation already demoralized by inaccuracy.'

This sociological understanding of punning by actors with schizophrenia can be supported both with other examples and with reference to other theorists. For instance, Torrey cites the following exchange between himself and a patient. 'What would you do if you were lost in a forest?' Wherein lies the necessity of this question? The question 'What would you do if you were lost in a forest?' is problematic because the patient is already experiencing a certain kind of disorientation. Intersubjectively, the patient is lost in a forest of emotions and sense-perceptions. Does it matter to the patient if one were hypothetically lost in a forest? Wherein lies the reality of the physician's question in so far as the reality of the question resides in the relation between the physician and patient as a dialogical relation? The necessity of this question resides in the right of science to make discoveries and inquiries with whatever means possible.

How does the patient reply to the question 'What would you do if you were lost in a forest?' The patient says, 'Go to the back of the forest, not the front.' From a physician's point of view, the answer is symptomatic. From a sociological point of view, the patient takes the falseness of the physician's question and transforms it into an illusion of truth, an illusion of truth that in its literalness traps the falseness of the physician's question. Foucault describes the process this way: 'Madness is the purest, most total form of *quid pro quo*.'[31]

Let us consider another example. In *Is There No Place on Earth for Me?*, Susan Sheehan reports Silvia as saying, 'Adolf Hitler is forgiven. He invented methadone and the Mercedes-Benz. It was all a prize war.' What is it for Sylvia to make this statement? Is the Holocaust something to laugh about? What does it mean for a young Jewish woman with schizophrenia to make this statement? Are the signifiers – Hitler, methadone, and a Mercedes-Benz – arbitrary in their ordering? Are the signifiers random in their interconnectedness?

From a Jewish point of view, 'we must never forget'; such is the prevailing order. To forgive Hitler transgresses the principle of modern Jewish identity, and an important aspect of who Sylvia is is her family's heritage and survival of the Second World War. If an ironic relation to the Holocaust is taboo, why is it taboo? What does it mean then for Silvia to say, 'Adolf Hitler is forgiven. He invented methadone and the Mercedes-Benz. It was all a prize war'? Is she making a pun? Is there anti-Semitism in her statement? Is Sylvia doing a parody of anti-Semitism as a way to defend herself from anti-Semitism?[32] Is the weight of anti-Semitism for Sylvia an insignificant weight compared with what it means to suffer schizophrenia?

Jean-Paul Sartre writes: 'The anti-Semites have the *right* to play. They even like to play with discourse for, by giving ridiculous reasons, they discredit the seriousness of their interlocutors.'[33] Is the play of someone with schizophrenia like the play of the anti-Semite? Does Sylvia wish to discredit the seriousness of her interlocutor, in this case, Susan Sheehan, by giving ridiculous reasons? How is the play of someone with schizophrenia like but also unlike the play of the anti-Semite which Sartre describes? Why is the play of the anti-Semite, or any demagogue for that matter, more tolerated? Why do people find the play of the demagogue attractive and riveting and the play of someone with schizophrenia repellant?

We need a theorist like Foucault to glimpse the importance of what Sylvia is doing – 'Madness deals not so much with truth and the world, as with man and whatever truth about himself he is able to perceive.'[34] It is time to address the subject of motivation in the action of people with schizophrenia.

6

ACTION

Max Weber, R.D. Laing, and G.W.F. Hegel

We come now to the last step in our analysis of inner planes of verbal thought. Thought is not the superior authority in this process. Thought is not begotten by thought; it is engendered by motivation, i.e., by our desires and needs, our interests and emotions. Behind every thought there is an affective-volitional tendency, which holds the answer to the last 'why' in the analysis of thinking. A true and full understanding of another's thought is possible only when we understand its affective-volitional basis.

                                                          – Lev Vygotsky[1]

Schizophrenia is a troublesome phenomenon. It generates significant problems in social understanding and interpersonal relations. Medical research has made persuasive advances in the empirical treatment of schizophrenia, but social science has yet to construct (with any sort of theoretical confidence) what Max Weber would call 'an adequately meaningful level of understanding.' In his discussion of causal explanations and their place in the theory construction of the social sciences, Weber warns:

If adequacy in respect to meaning is lacking, then no matter how high the degree of uniformity and how precisely its probability can be numerically determined, it is still an incomprehensible statistical probability, whether dealing with overt or subjective processes.[2]

Is research heading towards such a situation with respect to schizophrenia? Is it possible to have a causal explanation of a phenomenon without adequately understanding the meaningfulness of that phenomenon for which we have a causal explanation?

One of the frightening aspects of schizophrenia is that it reminds us that the brain, which is, let us say, the 'house' of the mind, is a natural phenomenon and, as such, is subject to the laws of organic nature. This feature of schizophrenia makes it hard to accept schizophrenia as an illness. It is easier to accept a broken arm than a damaged brain. The difficulty has to do with who we are as human beings. The mind functions independently of the brain.[3] We assume (call it hubris) that, even if the brain is dysfunctional, the mind ought to function well. We are disturbed when such is not the case. We are also disturbed when such is the case. Our notion of who we are as human beings is confronted. What is it about us that is independent of 'the physiological organism proper'?[4]

Before the onslaught of schizophrenia, the person had a self, exemplified self-consciousness, and engaged in social action. Why would we stop viewing the person in these terms? After being diagnosed as 'schizophrenic,' and so labelled, the person retains his or her capacity for social action.

Schizophrenia is not a character flaw, but people with schizophrenia have character. Moreover, people with schizophrenia want their character (who and what they are as human beings) to be acknowledged and appreciated by others in social interaction.[5]

The documentary *Full of Sound and Fury*, sponsored by the Ontario Educational Communications Authority, makes this point clearly and eloquently. Unlike most documentaries, this one insists that people with schizophrenia be allowed to speak for themselves, and the documentary does so without being the least bit patronizing. The film respects the dignity and humanity of its subjects by allowing its narrative to be governed by people with schizophrenia. Often, documentaries have a narrator speak over top of the words of someone with schizophrenia. The message is that what the person with schizophrenia is saying is of no consequence to the film's audience. Tzvie, a subject in *Full of Sound and Fury* says:

I don't see why a schizophrenic can't be helped to achieve a status other than a ward of the state ... to be something more than just schizophrenic ... I'm not like other people, but I want to be something like other people, something like it ... I can't be altogether like it ... I want to be something like it and for me to lock myself away inside a closet and accept schizophrenic – I can't do that. It's cutting your throat without a knife.

Ideal Types

Research on schizophrenia is still controversial in some circles, but there is one point with which all would have to agree namely – that people with schizophrenia make choices that influence their lives and sense of selves. Even Nancy Andreason, the hard-core neurologist and author of *The Broken Brain*, expresses her agreement with this point when she remarks:

Living our lives with our own particular assigned brains is like playing a game of cards with a particular hand that we have been dealt. We cannot control the cards we are given, but we can choose how we will play them.[6]

How do we choose the cards we play? Do the cards choose for us, or does something other than the cards govern how we play the hand? Is it the cards (the neurons in the brain) that determine the play of the hand, or something else? If it is something else (agency, motivation, will), how do we understand this aspect of action?

Lev Vygotsky says that 'the last why' in the analysis of thinking does not reside in thought. It resides in motivation. Thought does not engender thought; motivation does. (What motivation engenders the thought of science?)[7] With this point, Vygotsky asks sociology to come on the scene. The problem is that sociologists as scientists cannot establish causal explanations of motivation. This fact of life both animates and vexes sociological inquiry.

While sociologists cannot establish causal explanations of motivation, they can, Weber argues, establish adequately meaningful explanations of motivation. To explicate the motivation of a social action (the agency of the action), sociologists employ an ideal type, and Weber is categorical on this point.[8] To analyse social action in its entirety (its conditions, means, ends, normative orientation, agency) and to see the interdependence of each component, sociologists draw upon an ideal type, that does not itself fall within the domain of positivistic epistemology.[9] Sociologists need an ideal type to explicate the whole which is greater than the sum of the parts, which is not to say that the ideal type employed is itself the whole. The whole is always greater than the sum of the parts, including the part that is the ideal type, whose purpose is to explain the functional relation of the different parts. Here is how Talcott Parsons describes this inevitable feature of sociological inquiry:

The only positive characterization of the ideal type that Weber gives is that it is a construction of elements abstracted from the concrete, and put together to form a unified conceptual pattern. This involves a one-sided exaggeration (*Steigerung*) of certain aspects of the concrete reality, but is not to be found in it, that is, concretely existing, except in a few very special cases, such as purely rational action.[10]

Sociology does not need a special methodology to enlarge the parameters of social epistemology through which to understand schizophrenia as a human phenomenon. What is required is the same methodology which sociologists employ to study any instance of social action. Indeed, with no other subject is Weber's call for the use of ideal types more compelling. Schizophrenia challenges empirical study in the social as well as the natural sciences.

Have there been studies that employed an ideal type to analyse the motive-guided action of people with schizophrenia? There have been, but more often than not such studies have occurred outside of the realm of sociology. For instance, the goal of *The Divided Self* is not to provide causal explanations of schizophrenia, but, in Laing's own words, 'to make madness, and the process of going mad, comprehensible.'[11] Laing seeks to grasp schizophrenia empathetically through such notions as 'ontological insecurity' and 'divided self.' He asks after the logic with which the self-consciousness of someone with schizophrenia relates to the actuality that is schizophrenia. Laing's commitment is to 'Verstehen.'[12]

Laing's Reification

As noted in previous chapters, Torrey is highly critical of Laing's studies; he disparagingly refers to Laing's work as 'romantic nonsense devoid of any scientific basis.'[13] He says that Laing's theorizing is nothing more than 'theories-reified-as-facts.'[14] For Torrey, the error in Laing's work is that he treats the thing-like phenomenon that is schizophrenia as if it were, in and of itself, a concept, as if the essence of schizophrenia were the ontology of a metaphysical concept. For Torrey, schizophrenia has a thing-like quality subject to experimental methodology, and this is the only point for research on schizophrenia.[15]

When Torrey charges reification, he is saying that Laing 'fixes' the phenomenon of schizophrenia to a concept that is independent of the phenomenon itself.[16] It is worth asking, though, whether Laing reifies whatever concept that happens to come to him or if he, in fact, reifies one particular concept and, if so, which one?

I argue that there is one particular concept that Laing reifies when he examines schizophrenia, and this concept is what Hegel speaks of in *The Phenomenology of Mind* as 'The Unhappy Consciousness.' The Unhappy Consciousness is that strange and unhealthy marriage of Stoicism and Scepticism. In this chapter I support Torrey's charge of reification against Laing, but I theorize so as to defuse its purely polemical character.

What is the law, the logic, with which the self-consciousness of someone with schizophrenia relates to the actuality that is schizophrenia? To address this question, Laing employs the Unhappy Consciousness as an ideal type, and there is nothing wrong with such use of a concept. Weber maintains that it is necessary. As is well known, Marx draws upon Hegel's Master/Slave dialectic for his theory of class conflict. Weber argues: 'In *all* cases, rational or irrational ... analysis both abstracts from reality and at the same time helps us to understand it.'[17] To understand schizophrenia as a human reality, Laing employs a concept that is independent of that reality but which helps him to understand it. As an ideal type, the concept provides a adequacy on the level of meaning by virtue of its high degree of logical integration with the phenomenon. To protect such theorizing from the charge of reification, however, it is necessary to keep in mind Weber's caveat: 'it is probably seldom if ever that a real phenomenon can be found which corresponds exactly to one of these ideally constructed pure types.'[18] Laing's mistake is believing and arguing that schizophrenia is the Unhappy Consciousness. The question is: Can we preserve Laing's approach without making his mistake?

The Unhappy Consciousness

The following passage provides an exegesis of the Unhappy Consciousness and suggests its implicit correlation to schizophrenia:

Unable to exert effective influence on the extreme world, the 'Unhappy Consciousness' represents an oscillation between the cultivation of inner life directed toward an immutable abstract eternity and a continued but continuously frustrated interest in the affairs of the objective world.[19]

In light of this statement on what the Unhappy Consciousness is, consider the following account of what it is like to experience schizophrenia:

Things are coming in too fast. I lose my grip of it and get lost. I am attending to everything at once and as a result I do not really attend to anything.[20]

To give another example, consider Sandy's comments in *Full of Sound and Fury* on what it is like for her to be psychotic:

When I'm psychotic, I have no feeling in my body. I have no relation to my body. I feel like I'm a disembodied soul. I'm in contact with fairy kings, delusionary people. Sometimes I'm not even aware there are normal people around me. I'm so caught up in the fantasy and I think sometimes I thought I was Peter Rabbit and I would only eat rabbit food ... It's scary. It's very frightening and it's terrifying. And I can remember, too, once I thought that I was being punished by having bees swarm all over me and being stung and I felt that I was being stung and it was terrifying. It's real, it's not imaginary at the time.

What is the law, the logic, with which self-consciousness relates to the actuality that is schizophrenia? How is it that someone whose actuality is the experience of schizophrenia might adapt the Unhappy Consciousness as a viable and appropriate self-consciousness?

Speaking of Hegel's masterwork, Stanley Rosen says: 'The *Phenomenology* is the story of the connection between logic and appearance as that connection appears to the human spirit. As a 'story,' it is both a description and an interpretation.'[21] The Unhappy Consciousness is one chapter in Hegel's story, and it is a chapter that has significantly influenced Friedrich Nietzsche, Søren Kierkegaard, Martin Heidegger, and Jean-Paul Sartre. Postmodern theorists suggest that this one chapter represents the entire story of the human spirit. Even Rosen, who is not a postmodern thinker, oversimplifies when he writes: 'Wherever wisdom is absent there we find the unhappy consciousness.'[22] This statement is not correct because, for Hegel, there is a thread of wisdom in every chapter of the *Phenomenology*, even the one on the Unhappy Consciousness.

What then is this thread of wisdom that Hegel shows the Unhappy Consciousness grasping? This question is important because, in so far as someone with schizophrenia adapts the Unhappy Consciousness as an appropriate one for his or her actuality, the person grasps this thread of wisdom.[23]

When Laing 'sees' schizophrenia, he explains the 'logic' of that phenomenon as the logic of the Unhappy Consciousness. The preoccupation of the person with schizophrenia is to preserve, not his or her body, but his or her self-consciousness. The fear is the horror of a life without self-consciousness, the horror of failing to be an authentic member of one's species-being.[24]

In Hegel's analysis, the Unhappy Consciousness evolves from the self-consciousness of the Stoic and the Sceptic, and this development represents that thread of wisdom that is particular to the Unhappy Consciousness. The Stoic rejects the external world. The Stoic's non-relation to reality makes the Stoic free, but this freedom is abstract, and the Stoic is enslaved by this abstractness. While thoughtful, the Stoic lacks content, that is, a determinate relation to reality.[25]

The Sceptic appears on the scene *vis-à-vis* the Stoic by making the implicit negativity of the Stoic explicit, and thereby real. The Sceptic celebrates the Stoic's implied freedom through relentless negativity.[26] The problem is that, in negating the significance and determinateness of others, the Sceptic at the same time negates the significance and determinateness of the Sceptic.[27]

How, then, does the Unhappy Consciousness evolve from the limit of the Stoic and the Sceptic? The Stoic and the Sceptic, while opposites, are interrelated. The Unhappy Consciousness comes into existence in so far as Stoicism and Scepticism form one entity. Thus, when the Unhappy Consciousness is at peace with its inner nature, it is raging and at war with the external world – 'the Unhappy Sceptic.' When the Unhappy Consciousness is at war with itself, its inner nature, it is at peace with the external world – 'the Unhappy Stoic.' The dialectic of the Unhappy Consciousness is negative, but, when inverted, a positive content is disclosed. The Unhappy Consciousness is a self-consciousness that anticipates the horror of a life without self-consciousness.

The Unhappy Consciousness cures itself; that is, it *in itself* develops, when it grasps that thread of wisdom which is itself, when it comes to see the unity of Stoicism and Scepticism as its particular essence. Here is the knowledge of the Unhappy Consciousness that grounds its particular wisdom *vis-à-vis* Stoicism and Scepticism, and for Hegel this is but one moment in the story of the human spirit as it constructs for itself the story of the connection between logic and appearance.

The Beautiful Soul

The Unhappy Consciousness, I stress, is a 'typical' way in which people with schizophrenia may interpret and understand the meaningfulness of their experience with schizophrenia.[28] It is only adequate with respect to meaning; it is neither categorical nor causal. Some people may interpret their experience with schizophrenia through another type of self-consciousness. For instance, some may understand and make sense of their actuality through the notion that Hegel calls 'the Beautiful Soul,' a concept developed later in the *Phenomenology*:

Conscience, then, in its majestic sublimity above any specific law and every content of duty, puts whatever content it pleases into its knowledge and willing. It is moral genius and originality, which knows the inner voice of its immediate knowledge to be a voice divine.[29]

This passage evokes the idea of the oracle. The action of the oracle is to put 'whatever content it pleases into its knowledge and willing' and it 'knows the inner voice of its immediate knowledge to be a voice divine.' The Beautiful Soul could be another self-consciousness with which to understand what it is to experience schizophrenia as a human being. One might even argue that the Beautiful Soul is a healthier form of self-consciousness for someone relating to the experience of schizophrenia.

Schizophrenia strikes people independently of class and level of intelligence. This point was dramatized recently when John Nash, the great economist from Princeton University who was diagnosed with schizophrenia in 1958 during the prime of his career (from a Freudian perspective) was awarded the Nobel Prize in economics in 1994, at the age of sixty-six. Nash's symptoms had gone into remission, and he was able to travel to Sweden to accept his award for his revolutionary work in game theory. As a mathematical genius afflicted with schizophrenia, Nash appears to have adopted during his suffering a self-consciousness that is like the one that Hegel describes as the Beautiful Soul. In *The New York Times*, Sylvia Nasar reports on Nash's life after having stepped down from his academic position:

There he became the Phantom of Fine Hall, a mute figure who scribbled strange equations on blackboards in the mathematics building and searched anxiously for secret messages in numbers.[30]

Nasar also writes:

Alicia Nash [Nash's wife] believed very firmly, according to several people close to her, that Mr. Nash should live at home and stay within Princeton's mathematics community even when he was not functioning well. 'Being in Princeton was good for him,' said Mrs. Legg [Nash's sister]. 'In a place like Princeton, if you act strange, you're special. In Roanoke [Mr. Nash's childhood home in Virginia], if you act strange, you're just different. They didn't know who he was here.'

Roger Lewin, a psychiatrist in Baltimore, agrees. 'Some people are so disturbed that there is no way to get in touch with them, but for a significant group, compassion and receptivity of the surrounding community make all the difference.'[31]

Notice that there does not need to be an opposition between this study's 'restorative' reading of the existential–phenomenological understanding of schizophrenia and the biological understanding. When the brain (for whatever reason or cause) is afflicted with the illness that is called schizophrenia, the logic of necessity grips the mind with a particular self-consciousness. That self-consciousness might be the Unhappy Consciousness, and it might not. There is no attempt here to generate a causal explanation; the interest is phenomenological – to grasp the logic of the experience of schizophrenia for the self-conscious human being.

Here is the lesson of the Unhappy Consciousness, and some with schizophrenia teach it very well. How does self-consciousness exist within the empirical world as a non-empirical existence? The problem (and it is a problem for every human being whose spirit seeks wisdom) is to grasp self-consciousness as an entity that is real but non-empirical. If self-consciousness has an empirical existence, self-consciousness *qua* self-consciousness is non-existent. (It is a thing.) If self-consciousness has a non-empirical existence, self-consciousness *qua* self-consciousness is also non-existent. (It is unreal, that is, metaphysical.)

The Unhappy Consciousness cures itself; that is, it develops, when it comes to know, not its detachment, but its autonomy *vis-à-vis* reality. Autonomy is self-consciousness being aware of its existence in the empirical world as a non-empirical entity; autonomy sustains the objectivity of self-consciousness where objectivity now is something quite different from being empirically correct.

But Hegel, as he always does, qualifies this achievement in the following way: For the self-consciousness that emancipates itself from the Unhappy Consciousness, autonomy is neither the direct object of action (the mistake of Scepticism) nor the fundamental principle of action (the limit of Stoicism).[32] Autonomy is a resource for action and the principled development of the human spirit, and it is a resource that people with schizophrenia vehemently fight to retain. In drawing upon Hegel's notion of the Unhappy Consciousness, whether consciously or not, Laing grasps, at an explanatory level, the mind's struggle with the illness that is schizophrenia, and it is a struggle with which we all can empathize and from which we all can learn.[33]

To note an example: in *Full of Sound and Fury* Sandy says to the camera:

I have something to offer society. It may not be as much as the next guy, but I feel my contribution is valuable and I want to offer it when I can. There are times when I can't ... when I'm sick and I have to be in the hospital. But when I'm well, I have something I want to give. I want to be part of the world.

Laing, of course, also employs Hegel's Master/Slave dialectic as an ideal type in his analysis of schizophrenia. The tension between the true self and the false self, the healthy self and the unhealthy self, is the tension of the Master/Slave dialectic recast in an individual context. The problem of the divided self is that the false self *qua* Master oppresses the true self *qua* Slave, and recovery is analogous to the emancipation of the true self from the tyranny of the false self. Laing draws upon the Master/Slave dialectic for his analysis of the divided self and the problem of authencity.

My argument is that, while Laing's use of the Master/Slave dialectic is a manifest one, his use of the Unhappy Consciousness is a latent one. Moreover, Laing's latent use of the Unhappy Consciousness is more critical for understanding schizophrenia than Laing's manifest use of the Master/Slave dialectic. Laing's analysis of the tension between the true self and the false self, however enlightening, does not contribute directly to the explication of schizophrenia. All people (those with schizophrenia and those not) exemplify an interplay and interdependence between their false selves and their true selves. Schizophrenia is not a psychoanalytical problem, but, at the same time, people with schizophrenia may have psychoanalytical problems which (in and of themselves) have no causal relation to schizophrenia.

For instance, people with schizophrenia, like Sandy and Tzvie, may free themselves from their false selves and the oppression of inauthenticity but continue to be diagnosed 'schizophrenic.' That is, people with schizophrenia may come to know their true selves as much as is humanly possible and still suffer schizophrenia. Indeed, by virtue of having suffered and placed the affliction called 'schizophrenia,' people may become wise. Likewise, people who have not suffered schizophrenia may never come to free themselves from their false selves so as to embrace their true selves and a sense of authenticity.

EPILOGUE

Beyond Altruism

It is a selfish society that only assumes responsibility for what it understands to be its direct effects, as if poverty were such an effect and blindness were not. Imagine a society that only took responsibility for the effects it understood itself to have created rather than for those in its midst who suffered any sort of injustice. Research on disability does not do the disabled a favour by saying: 'Well that's your problem, but I will help you out of the kindness of my heart.' Rather, research says: 'The suffering of all within my midst is my problem because society means an oriented readiness to respond thoughtfully to the injustice of suffering.

– Alan Blum[1]

There would seem then to be not merely a separation of egoism and rationality ... but a reverse connection, with increasing rationality man becomes less rather than more egoistic.

– Talcott Parsons[2]

Readers may ask what experiences I have and what studies I engaged in to write this book. The evidence in this work is not governed by conventional notions of empirical inquiry. Rather than cite experimentally determined data that I or someone else has generated, I draw upon examples from first-person accounts, biographies, clinical reports, news reports, and film documentaries. The justification for this dependency resides in part on Talcott Parsons's insistence that, in sociological inquiry, a fact never speaks for itself. In sociology, a fact is not really a fact. A fact is a statement, and so itself an icon grounded in a perspective, ideology, or value commitment.[3] The task is not to list every fact which surrounds a subject but to formulate and account for why a certain set of facts is deemed significant. From a theoretical point of view, the material used in this study is as useful and as compelling as any experimentally determined data that I or someone else might have generated.

Still, it is often said that theorists do their best work when engaged with some empirical phenomenon. In deference to this truism, I would like to close with a talk that I gave while working as a volunteer with a schizophrenic population on a locked ward at Queen Street Mental Health Centre in Toronto, Ontario. The experience described in this talk motivated me eventually to design and teach a university course titled 'Schizophrenia and Social Science.' Teaching this course emboldened me to start publishing articles on schizophrenia in social science journals and to write this book. I continue to engage in volunteer activities in my present community with people afflicted with schizophrenia.

I have been doing volunteer work at the Queen Street Mental Health Centre in Toronto for two years. I work with adult patients who are diagnosed with chronic schizophrenia. Once a week, on Thursday evenings, another volunteer and I initiate and run a bingo game for about two hours. Usually ten to twenty patients participate.

The game of bingo, I discovered, is a very acceptable and enjoyable activity for the people participating, especially if we keep the game simple by playing one line rather than two lines, four corners, the whole card, or 'T.' Bingo is a game in which many people can participate and in which nobody feels that his or her performance is on the line. The game is not stressful because the player does not have to make any practical or calculated decisions while playing. The player hears the number and places the appropriate chip on the card, and for the schizophrenic patient this task can be enough of a challenge. Game prizes, which the Queen Street Volunteer Association provides, are either cigarettes or candy.

At the time that I decided to start doing volunteer work in a mental health centre, I was close to completing my doctoral dissertation in sociology and was waiting to start a teaching assignment. I was impressed by the fact that the Queen Street Mental Health Centre asked their volunteers to make a firm, six-month commitment. It made me realize that the centre took their volunteers seriously and considered the work of their volunteers to be important. In asking for this time commitment, the centre also demonstrated that they cared for and had concern for their patients.

After I became involved and saw the value and benefit of this work, I continued on. I saw that this experience was unique and could not be duplicated in another setting. To spend two hours in the evening with a group of patients who suffer from schizophrenia is an experience that is difficult to account for adequately. There were many things that occurred both between patients and between the patients and me; often I would not understand the significance of what happened, or if what happened was, in fact, significant.

While at times the interactions on the ward seemed eerie and unreal, after I left the medical centre, I would find that there were interactions in the normal, everyday world that were just as eerie and unreal. In turn, I often found the exchanges that I had with patients to be very real, meaningful, and quite touching. The person who suffers from schizophrenia is fully capable of responding to the goodwill of a volunteer as well as expressing his or her goodwill towards the volunteer.

There are advantages to being a volunteer. Although there are limits to your relation with the patient (the volunteer is neither a professional therapist nor a family member), these limits can provide a positive and constructive basis on which to build a significant relationship between you and the other. Basically, your relation is non-clinical, and the patients know this. They enjoy interacting with someone who is friendly and interested in them but who is not clinical-minded. Patients talk about themselves, gossip, ask about you, make jokes, and laugh at your jokes. People who suffer from schizophrenia appreciate the chance to be engaged with someone who is concerned about them but who is not explicitly involved in their therapeutic treatment. Patients can be open with a volunteer without the fear of being diagnosed or tested.

Although the volunteer's relation is non-clinical, it is important for the volunteer to be responsible. For example, it is important for volunteers to come on time because the patients look forward to the bingo game and are in fact waiting in anticipation. For many this activity provides a healthy escape from the oppressive ennui of the ward. Patients feel disappointed if a volunteer is late, and they express this disappointment, sometimes by refusing to play.

It is also important for the volunteer to be consistent and fair in the way that the bingo game is run. Patients are very sensitive to any favouritism or inconsistencies. It is necessary for the volunteer to limit the effects of any aggressive behaviour that will undermine the group activity. The patients appreciate your firmness towards aggressive patients who, in my experience, often tended to be non-schizophrenic patients from other floors.

What a volunteer does for the mental health patient is to provide a bridge between the world of the mental health centre and the outside. With a volunteer, patients can share themselves, and share their life on the ward with someone from outside that world. In sharing themselves, patients get to 'leave' the ward, to establish space between themselves and their immediate relation to that medical world in which they live. In other words, with a volunteer, a person who suffers from schizophrenia gets the chance to be a non-patient, to be the very person who he or she is.

In the evening the atmosphere on the ward is more relaxed. Patients are not expecting anything. There is no rigorous agenda with which they are expected to comply. Therapists and psychiatrists are away for the evening, and so patients gain more space and are in fact in more control of their environment. They have more autonomy, which is a luxury for some and a horror for others.

When I first started doing volunteer work, I thought of myself as fairly independent from the psychiatrist and the medical staff. I came during the evening and I enjoyed this independence. But I came to realize that the professional team with which I worked was very interested in hearing about our experiences and observations through a communication book that they left at the nurses' station for volunteers. The team made it clear that they knew we were getting to know the people on their ward in a way that they often could not; they liked to hear about our experiences because it was helpful to them in their understanding and treatment of their patients. By sharing our experiences and thoughts through the communication book, I came to feel that we were helping, both directly and indirectly, the people whom we were getting to know. We were helping to build a bridge, a human bridge over which people with schizophrenia could cross from the isolated community of the mental health centre to the outside world called 'society,' of which they are already a part.[4]

Notes

PROLOGUE

1 *Toward a Rational Society: Student Protest, Science, and Politics* (Boston: Beacon Press 1968), 61.
2 Today causal explanations of schizophrenia are the exclusive domain of neurology. The 'nature' rather than 'nurture' explanation of schizophrenia is the hegemonic one in medical research and health care, although there have been some reconsiderations of social variables from within the purview of the neurological explanation. See E. Fuller Torrey, *Surviving Schizophrenia: A Family Manual*, rev. ed. (New York: Harper & Row 1988); Nancy C. Andreason, *The Broken Brain: The Biological Revolution in Psychiatry* (New York: Harper & Row 1984); and, for reconsiderations of social variables by a neurologist, Irving I. Gottesman, *Schizophrenia Genesis: The Origins of Madness* (New York: W.H. Freeman and Company 1991).
3 See Schizophrenia Research Branch, *Schizophrenia: Questions and Answers* (Rockville, MD: National Institute of Mental Health 1986).
4 'What Is Schizophrenia?' in *Schizophrenia Digest* 2 (January 1995), 4. The article notes that 'Canada spends $4 billion a year to support sick individuals, in and out of hospitals.'
5 Talcott Parsons, *The Social System* (Glencoe: Free Press 1951), 431.
6 For an example of another sociological theorist who takes this position, see Peter Barham, *Schizophrenia and Human Value* (London: Free Association Books 1993).
7 Parsons, *The Social System*, 436.
8 For a defence from within the tradition of sociology of this dualistic under-

standing of the human being, see Emile Durkheim's 'The Dualism of Human Nature and Its Social Consequences,' where Durkheim, the great empiricist, writes: 'Thus the traditional antithesis of the body and soul is not a vain mythological concept that is without foundation in reality. It is true that we are double, that we are the realization of an antimony' (*Emile Durkheim*, edited by Kurt H. Wolff [New York: Arno Press 1979], 329–30).

CHAPTER ONE

1 *The Broken Brain: The Biological Revolution in Psychiatry* (New York: Harper & Row 1984), 83. This chapter is a revision of my article 'Mead's Theory of Self and Schizophrenia,' *Social Science Journal* 29 (1992), 307–21.
2 E. Fuller Torrey, *Surviving Schizophrenia: A Family Manual*, rev. ed. (New York: Harper & Row 1988), 17.
3 George Herbert Mead, *Mind, Self, and Society* (Chicago: University of Chicago Press 1934).
4 See Charles Cooley's classic essay 'Sympathy or Understanding as an Aspect of Society,' in *Human Nature and the Social Order* (New York: Scribner's 1922), 136–67.
5 Torrey, *Surviving Schizophrenia*, 286.
6 John S. Strauss, 'Subjective Experiences of Schizophrenia: Toward a New Dynamic Psychiatry – II,' *Schizophrenia Bulletin* 15 (1989), 179–86. Think here of Max Weber, who writes: 'Action is social in so far as, by virtue of the subjective meaning attached to it by the acting individual (or individuals), it takes account of the behavior of others and is thereby oriented in its course' (in *The Theory of Social and Economic Organization* [New York: Free Press 1947], 88).
7 Strauss, 'Subjective Experiences of Schizophrenia,' 182.
8 See Jaber F. Gubrium, 'The Social Preservation of Mind: The Alzheimer's Disease Experience,' *Symbolic Interaction* 8 (1986), 37–51. I was influenced by Gubrium's thoughtful use of Mead's work for the construction of a social understanding of Alzheimer's disease, but, as Mead notes, 'the unity of the mind is not identical with the unity of the self' (*Mind, Self and Society*, 144). For example, psychiatrists distinguish a patient with schizophrenia from one with brain damage with the diagnostic observation that the one with schizophrenia is 'oriented.' 'A patient was considered "oriented times three" if he knew (1) who he was, (2) where he was, and (3) what day it was. Schizophrenics are usually oriented, which helps distinguish them from patients with brain damage': Carol North, *Welcome, Silence* (New York: Avon Books 1987), 8. That a patient may be delusional but 'oriented' exemplifies what Mead discusses as the difference between mind and self.

9 North, *Welcome, Silence*; Marguerite Sechehaye, *Autobiography of a Schizo-phrenic Girl* (New York: Signet 1951); Susan Sheehan, *Is There No Place on Earth for Me?* (New York: Vintage Books 1983).

10 Mead, *Mind, Self, and Society,* 136.

11 People afflicted with schizophrenia are today's pariahs, which is why post-modern thinkers like Jacques Lacan and Gilles Deleuze find the subject of schizophrenia so appealing for their theorizing. For Lacan and Deleuze, schizophrenia (as a social rather than a physical phenomenon) becomes an ideal, heuristic vehicle for their intellectualizing; that is, as social actors, peo-ple with schizophrenia appear to stand beyond the realm of rationality, not unlike the very theorizing of postmodernism itself. In other words, 'the fig-ure of the schizophrenic' comes to stand as the postmodernist's theoretic hero. See Alphonse De Waelhens, *Schizophrenia: A Philosophical Reflection on Lacan's Structuralist Interpretation,* translated by W. Ver Eecke (Pittsburgh: Duquesne University Press 1978), and Gilles Deleuze and Félix Guattari, *Anti-Oedipus: Capitalism and Schizophrenia* (Minneapolis: University of Min-nesota Press 1983).

12 Torrey, *Surviving Schizophrenia,* 65.

13 Nancy Andreason, an authority on the neurological understanding of schizo-phrenia, writes from a strong positivistic perspective: 'While the brain is something that can be seen, felt, and studied under a miscroscope, the mind is an abstract concept that usually refers to the activities the brain generates' (*The Broken Brain,* 21). See Jeff Coulter's 'The Brain as Agent,' *Human Studies* 2 (1979), 335–48.

14 Sheehan, *Is There No Place on Earth for Me?,* 243.

15 R.D. Laing makes a poignant use of the Meadian distinction 'I' and 'me' to account for the troubled self of someone with schizophrenia when he writes: 'There is still an "I" that cannot find a "me." An "I" has not ceased to exist, but it is without substance, it is disembodied, it lacks the quality of realness, and it has no identity, it has no "me" to go with it. It may seem a contradic-tion in terms to say that the "I" lacks identity but this seems to be so. The schizophrenic either does not know who or what he is or he has become something or someone other than himself. At any rate, without such a last shred or scrap of a self, an "I" therapy of any kind would be impossible' (*The Divided Self* [Harmonsworth: Penguin 1969], 172).

The self of someone with schizophrenia can thus be seen to be divided in two Meadian senses: the self from its body and the 'I' from its 'me.' While inspired by Laing's work, this study differs by showing how the self with schizophrenia does not lose its 'me' to the degree that Laing indicates. The problem is not a psychoanalytic one. This matter is discussed more fully in chapter 4.

16 Mead, *Mind, Self, and Society,* 136.
17 Sechehaye, *Autobiography of a Schizophrenic Girl,* 58–9.
18 See Erving Goffman, 'The Moral Career of the Mental Patient,' in *Deviance: The Interactionist Perspective,* 3d ed., edited by Earl Rubington and Martin S. Weinberg (New York: Macmillan, 1978), 120–30; Harold Sampson, Sheldon L. Messinger, and Robert D. Towne, 'Family Processes and Becoming a Mental Patient,' in ibid., 46–55; and Edwin M. Lemert, 'Paranoia and the Dynamics of Exclusion,' in ibid., 131–40.
19 Mead, *Mind, Self, and Society,* 136.
20 Karl Marx, 'Alienated Labor,' *Karl Marx: Early Writings,* translated by T.B. Bottomore (New York: McGraw-Hill 1963), 125–7. 'The animal ... does not distinguish the activity from itself. It is its activity.' Marx differentiates the human being from the animal: 'But man makes his life activity itself an object of his will and consciousness. He has a conscious life activity ... Conscious life activity distinguishes man from the life activity of animals' (ibid.).
21 Sheehan, *Is There No Place on Earth for Me?,* 73.
22 Postmodern thinkers treat schizophrenia as a parody of society's inability to be reflexive, that is, of society and its members' inability to experience themselves as a whole. In other words, Deleuze and Lacan treat schizophrenia as a symbol, a mere symbol of the necessarily fragmented nature of social order. Kenneth Burke, an influential American literary critic and social theorist, identifies the problem and limit of a strictly 'literary' approach to social inquiry when he writes: 'I object ... to "symbolism" ... because it suggests too close a link with a particular school of poetry, the Symbolist Movement, and usually implies the unreality of the world in which we live, as though nothing could be what it is, but must always be something else' (*On Symbols and Society,* edited by J.R. Gusfield [Chicago: University of Chicago Press 1989], 79). As shown in chapter 4, the postmodern view of schizophrenia is non-epistemological and so, ironically enough, solely metaphysical. By way of contrast, the reductionist treatment of schizophrenia by clinical psychologists is merely epistemological, and lamentably non-metaphysical.

To clarify this point, it is helpful to mention here Martin Buber's I–Thou and I–It distinction where I–Thou is our relation to authentic, spiritual wholeness, and I–It our controlling relation to another as a thing or object. What does it mean to understand the actor with schizophrenia exclusively in terms of an I–It relation? Why is the actor with schizophrenia denied the privileged relation of I–Thou? Could not this actor be more open to the I–Thou relation and the non-schizophrenic in turn more open to the I–Thou relation in the very seeking to understand another human being suffering schizophrenia? See Martin Buber, *I and Thou* (New York: Collier Books 1987).

23 Sechehaye, *Autobiography of a Schizophrenic Girl*, 52–3. 'System' is a buzz word for the effects of schizophrenia on Renee's mind.

24 Torrey's chapter 'What the Family Needs,' in *Surviving Schizophrenia*, provides good practical advice and information in this regard, although Torrey does not formulate the sociological foundation for the positive character of his advice or how the basis for his advice differs from the neurological understanding of schizophrenia that he himself advocates (273–314): 'In general, the people who get along best with schizophrenics are those who treat them most naturally as people. This can be verified by watching the nursing staff in any psychiatric hospital. The staff who are most respected by both professionals and patients treat patients with dignity and as human beings, albeit with a brain disease' (284). For further discussion, see note 36.

25 Mead, *Mind, Self, and Society*, 172.

26 Ibid.

27 Torrey, *Surviving Schizophrenia*, 53–4.

28 Torrey writes: 'Dr. M.B. Rosenbaum, in a sensitive article on the sexual problems of persons with schizophrenia, described one patient who "vividly described all the angels and devils in his bedroom telling him what and what not to do while having intercourse"' (ibid., 258).

29 Mead, *Mind, Self, and Society*, 156.

30 Torrey, *Surviving Schizophrenia*, 57.

31 Mead, *Mind, Self, and Society*, 254.

32 See Ralph Turner, 'Role-Taking: Process versus Conformity,' in *Human Behavior and Social Processes*, edited by Arnold M. Rose (Boston: Houghton-Mifflin 1962), 20–40.

33 North, *Welcome, Silence*, 220.

34 Ibid., 221.

35 Erving Goffman, *The Presentation of Self in Everyday Life* (Garden City, NY: Doubleday Anchor Books 1959), 106–40.

36. Torrey's discussion of 'the disease trap,' where the person seems to merge completely with the sick role such that the two become indistinguishable from the viewpoint of, not only the family, but also the person with schizophrenia, is an interesting variation of this point. On this topic of role–person merger, see Ralph Turner's 'The Role and the Person,' *American Journal of Sociology* 84 (1978), 1–23. To deal with this problem, Torrey recommends: 'Resist the temptation to blame everything on schizophrenia and ask how many mistakes *you* made in the last week,' that is, for purposes of social understanding distinguish between the person and the disease (*Surviving Schizophrenia*, 288). Notice, however, that Torrey, like Andreason, exemplifies a crude form of positivism when he continues: 'Allow individuals with

schizophrenia to have a bad day now and then, just as we allow those of us
without schizophrenia to have a bad day. We all need such days since our
neurochemical and neurophysiological machinery does not work perfectly
all the time; extending the privilege of a bad day to individuals with schizophrenia is both common sense and common courtesy' (288–9). Is the foundation for the authority of common sense and common courtesy our
neurochemical and neurophysiological machinery?

37 North, *Welcome, Silence*, 88.
38 Ibid., 25.
39 Ibid., 25–6.
40 G.W.F. Hegel, 'Sense-Certainty, This, and Meaning,' in *The Phenomenology of
   Mind*, translated by J.B. Baille (Atlantic Highlands, NJ: Humanities Press
   1977), 149–60.
41 For a discussion of this epistemology and its significance to the problem of
   social understanding, see my article, 'The Person and the Limit of Empiri-
   cism,' *The Personalist Forum* 10 (Summer 1994), 1–13.
42 Mead, *Mind, Self, and Society*, 254.
43 Sechehaye, *Autobiography of a Schizophrenic Girl*, 23.
44 To justify this exaggeration, see Max Weber's discussion of the necessary use
   of ideal types in theoretical social inquiry (*The Theory of Social and Economic
   Organization*, 86–112).
45 The ideology which informs the intepretations and analysis in this book can
   be characterized as critical humanism. Paulo Freire writes: 'The real human-
   ist can be identified more by his trust in the people, which engages him in
   their struggle, than by a thousand actions in their favor without that trust'
   (*Pedagogy of the Oppressed* [New York: Continuum 1989], 47).
46 Mead, *Mind, Self, and Society*, 138–9.
47 Andreason is strikingly positivistic in her writing: 'The mind and the body
   are in fact inseparable. The word *mind* refers to those functions of the body
   that reside in the brain' (*The Broken Brain*, 219).
48 Sechehaye, *Autobiography of a Schizophrenic Girl*, 114.
49 Ibid., 120–1.

CHAPTER TWO

1 *Mental Illness and Psychology* (Berkeley: University of California Press 1987), 45.
   This chapter is a revision and synthesis of two of my articles: 'A Sociological
   Hermeneutics for Schizophrenic Language,' *Social Science Journal* 31/2 (1994),
   111–25, and 'A Burkean Hermeneutics for Understanding the Social Character
   of Schizophrenic Language,' *Symbolic Interaction* 17/2 (1994), 129–46.

2 Kenneth Burke, 'Semantic and Poetic Meaning,' in *The Philosophy of Literary Form* (Berkeley: University of California Press 1973), 141. For a complete listing of Burke's writing and a discussion of Burke's influence on sociology, see Kenneth Burke, *On Symbols and Society*, edited and with an introduction by Joseph R. Gusfield (Chicago: University of Chicago Press 1989).

3 Burke, 'Semantic and Poetic Meaning,' 150.

4 Ibid., 144.

5 My interpretive methodology in this chapter is Burkean as described in this passage: 'Hence, for the validity of "poetic" meanings, I should suggest that the "test" cannot be a formal one, as with the diagrams for testing a syllogism. Poetic characterizations do not categorically exclude each other in the either-true-or-false sense ... The test of a metaphor's validity is of a much more arduous sort, requiring nothing less than the *filling-out, by concrete body, of the characterizations which one would test*. There is no formal procedure (ibid., 145).

6 Carol North, *Welcome, Silence* (New York: Avon Books 1989), 137.

7 Sullivan writes: 'The beauty of written language and, in some degree, the charm of spoken language consist not in anything inherent in linguistic processes or language symbols, but in the fact that in our learning of language, in our observance of language behavior, and in our successful formulation of foresights to impress if not to intimidate our teachers, our wives, and our friends, we are depending on that group processes which I call "consensual validation"' ('The Language of Schizophrenia,' in *Language and Thought in Schizophrenia*, edited by J.S. Kasanin [New York: Norton 1964], 13).

8 In *Surviving Schizophrenia: A Family Manual*, rev. ed. (New York: Harper & Row 1988), E. Fuller Torrey uses an *ad hominem* argument to dissuade readers from either looking at or taking seriously Sullivan's writing: 'Sullivan was enamored with Freud's theory that failure of attachment to the mother in childhood led to unconscious homosexuality and paranoid schizophrenia; Sullivan himself was "dominated by an unhappy, indulgent mother," was "a homosexual who wished to be a heterosexual," and almost certainly experienced multiple episodes of schizophrenia' (162).

I understand Torrey's need to protect innocent families with siblings afflicted with schizophrenia from suffering the unnecessary guilt that is caused by misinformation on what schizophrenia is, but I do not endorse the means with which Torrey provides this protection. There are better ways to do a critique than with an *ad hominem* argument.

9 Marquerite Sechehaye, *Autobiography of a Schizophrenic Girl* (New York: Signet 1979), 135–6.

10 Burke, *On Symbols and Society*, 60.

11 While 'metaphor,' Bateson writes, 'is an indispensable tool of thought and expression – a characteristic of all human communication, even of that of the scientist, ... the peculiarity of the schizophrenic is not that he uses metaphors, but that he uses unlabelled metaphors': 'Toward a Theory of Schizophrenia,' with Don D. Jackson, Jay Haley, and John Weakland, in *Steps to an Ecology of Mind: Collected Essays in Anthropology, Psychiatry, Evolution, and Epistemology* by Gregory Bateson (San Francisco: Chadler 1972), 205.

12 Given the positivistic ideology that undergirds today's research on schizophrenia, work such as Bateson's is now portrayed in a very negative light. In a section titled 'Discarded Theories,' Torrey writes on the double-bind theory: 'The lead author of the original paper describing this theory was Gregory Bateson, an anthropologist who had undergone Jungian psychoanalysis ... the inspiration for the 'double-bind' came from his studies of communications theory, cybernetics, rituals among natives in Papua New Guinea, the communications of dolphins, and Lewis Carroll's *Through the Looking Glass*. No control studies were done and Bateson freely acknowledged that "this hypothesis has not been statistically tested." In fact it never was, and in retrospect the single most important antecedent of the theory appears to have been the thinking of Lewis Carroll' (*Surviving Schizophrenia*, 164). Torrey is mocking Bateson's theorizing on schizophrenia. While I acknowledge Torrey's description of the negative status of the double-bind theory as a causal explanation, I do not respect Torrey's use of sarcasm to evaluate another's work.

13 The advantages of the new drug clozapine can be great for people afflicted with schizophrenia. The risks, however, are also great. For instance, the video *Into Madness*, by Alan and Susan Raymond (1989), reports that Bob, who had enjoyed long walks up and down the aisles of a Kmart store, lost his sense of balance and coordination upon taking clozapine. Bob's loss was that he could no longer walk. Another, even more serious drawback of this medication is the possible development of agranulocytosis, a blood disease. *Time* reported that 'six of the 20,000 Americans who have been treated with clozapine have died from the condition' (Claudia Wallis and James Willwerth, 'Awakenings, Schizophrenia, A New Drug Brings Patients Back to Life,' *Time*, 6 July 1992, 53–5).

14 Torrey, *Surviving Schizophrenia*, 33.

15 Harold Garfinkel, *Studies in Ethnomethodology* (Englewood Cliffs, NJ: Prentice-Hall 1967), 76–103.

16 Torrey, *Surviving Schizophrenia*, 34.

17 Erving Goffman, *The Presentation of Self in Everyday Life* (Garden City, NY: Doubleday Anchor 1959), 148.

18 Garfinkel demonstrates that 'various considerations dictate that common understandings cannot possibly consist of a measured amount of shared agreement among persons on certain topics': *Studies in Ethnomethodolgy*, 38.

19 Norman Cameron, 'Reason, Regression and Communication in Schizophrenics,' in *Psychological Monographs*, edited John F. Dashiell, vol. 50, no. 1 (Columbus, OH: American Psychological Association 1938), 14–27 *passim*.

20 Roy H. Wolcott, 'Schizophrenese: A Private Language,' *Journal of Health and Social Behavior* 11 (1970),133.

21 Susan Baur, *The Dinosaur Man: Tales of Madness and Enchantment from the Backward* (New York: Harper Perennial 1991), 73.

22 Ibid., 82–3.

23 Ibid.

24 Albert Cohen defines reaction formation the following way in his studies of deviance: 'They "stand it on its head"; they exalt its opposition; they engage in malicious, spiteful, "ornery" behavior of all sorts to demonstrate not only to others, but to themselves as well, their contempt for the game they have rejected' (*Deviance and Control* [Englewood Cliffs, NJ: Prentice-Hall 1966], 66).

25 Bateson, 'Toward a Theory of Schizophrenia,' 205.

26 Ibid., 209.

27 Goffman, *The Presentation of Self in Everyday Life*, 50.

28 For a thoughtful study of this notable artist with schizophrenia, see Stephen A. Martin, 'Martin Ramirez: Psychological Hero,' *The Arts in Psychotherapy* 15 (1988), 189–205.

29 R.D. Laing, *The Divided Self* (Harmondsworth: Penguin 1969), 164.

30 Torrey, *Surviving Schizophrenia*, 165–8.

31 Laing, *The Divided Self*, 22–3.

32 Morris Rosenberg, *The Unread Mind: Unraveling the Mystery of Madness* (New York: Lexington Books 1992).

CHAPTER THREE

1 *Schizophrenia and Human Value* (London: Free Association Books 1993), 169. Some key points in this chapter were initially worked out in my article with Maureen Leonard, Laura Muhlenbruck, Sherry Teerlink, and Dana Vinyard: "mother is not holding competely respect": Making Social Sense of Schizophrenic Writing,' *Human Studies* 18 (1995), 89–106.

2 R.L. Rosenhan, 'Being Sane in Insane Places,' *Science* 179 (1973), 252.

3 Ibid.

4 Rosenhan cites hospital patients as commenting to psuedo-patients: 'You're not crazy. You're a journalist, or a professor [referring to the continual note-

taking]. You're checking up on the hospital.' While most of the patients were reassured by the pseudopatient's insistence that he had been sick before he came in but was fine now, some continued to believe that the pseudopatient was sane throughout hospitalization' (ibid., 252).

5 Erving Goffman, *The Presentation of Self in Everyday Life* (Garden City, NY: Doubleday Anchor 1959), 151.

6 Rosenhan, 'Being Sane in Insance Places,' 258.

7 Morris Rosenberg writes: 'Role-taking carries with it enormous social and personal benefits. As Flavell notes, role-taking allows genuine, rather than apparent, interaction; it permits cooperation, compromise, real argument; and it permits a depth of interpersonal relations otherwise unattainable' ('A Symbolic Interactionist View of Psychosis,' *Journal of Health and Social Behavior* 25 [1984], 291).

8 In his book, Rosenberg writes: 'Mental illness represents a radical rupture of the bond connecting human beings to one another. It takes two to make a psychotic – an actor and an observer. The key to the mystery of insanity, I shall contend, is the phenomenon of role-taking failure' (*The Unread Mind: Unraveling the Mystery of Madness* [New York: Lexington Books 1992], x).

9 E. Fuller Torrey, *Surviving Schizophrenia: A Family Manual*, rev. ed. (New York: Harper & Row 1988), 33.

10 Rosenberg, 'A Symbolic Interactionist View of Psychosis,' 293.

11 Ibid., 290.

12 This phrase resonates with Alfred Schutz's account of the life-world and its significance to the phenomenological understanding of the social.

13 Physicians are aware of the importance of role-taking for effective relations between care-givers and those with schizophrenia. It is worth noting Torrey's observation again: 'The people who get along best with schizophrenics are those who treat them most naturally as people. This can be verified by watching the nursing staff in any psychiatric hospital. The staff who are most respected by both professionals and patients treat the patients with dignity and as human beings' (*Surviving Schizophrenia*, 284).

14 R.D. Laing, *The Divided Self* (Harmondsworth: Penguin 1969), 165.

15 On this matter Louis A. Sass writes: 'What seems so alienating about schizophrenics ... cannot be separated from the self-alienation felt by the patients themselves. But if this is so, it has the odd implication that the observer's alienation may not, in fact, indicate a total failure of empathy: it may be a *shared* alienation, a feeling evoked by accurate intuitions of what the patient is actually going through' (*Madness and Modernism* [New York: Basic Books 1992], 241).

16 Anne Deveson, *Tell Me I'm Here: One Family's Experience of Schizophrenia* (New

York: Penguin 1991), 255. Deveson poignantly recounts her relationship with her son and her struggle with his schizophrenia, which tragically led to his suicide. Indeed, the compelling character of the entire book is Deveson's ability to take the role of her son as an afflicted individual.

17 Talcott Parsons writes: 'Just as positivism eliminates the creative, voluntaristic character of action by dispensing with the analytical significance of values, and the other normative elements by making them epiphenomena, so idealism has the same effect for the opposite reason – idealism eliminates the reality of the obstacles to the realization of values' (*The Structure of Social Action* [New York: Free Press 1968], 446).

18 I thank Dr John Strauss and acknowledge his writing for making this point empirically and ethically clear.

19 Torrey, *Surviving Schizophrenia*, 71.

20 Ibid.

21 Ibid.

22 Rosenberg, 'A Symbolic Interactionist View of Pyschosis,' 294.

23 The significance of this point for sociological inquiry was stressed to me in the teaching of Peter McHugh in the Graduate Programme of Sociology, York University. Lev Vygotsky shows the truth of this position when he writes: 'From our point of view, the drive for the satisfaction of needs [internal motivation] and the drive for adaptation to reality [external conditions] cannot be considered separate from and opposed to each other. A need can be truly satisfied only through a certain adaptation to reality. Moreover, there is not such thing as adaptation for the sake of adaptation; it is always directed by needs' (*Thought and Language*, edited and translated by Eugenia Hanfmann and Gertrude Vakar [Cambridge, MA: MIT Press 1962], 21).

24 Rosenberg, *The Unread Mind*, 41–46.

25 Ibid.

26 Jean Piaget writes: 'Autistic thought is subconscious, which means that the aims it pursues and the problems it tries to solve are not present in consciousness; it is not adapted to reality, but creates for itself a dream world of imagination; it tends, not to establish truths, but so to satisfy desires, and it remains strictly individual and incommunicable as such by means of language' (*The Language and Thought of the Child* [London: Routledge & Kegan Paul 1971], 43). For many, this definition of autistic thought is an apt description of schizophrenic language.

27 Piaget, cited in Vygotsky, *Thought and Language*, 12.

28 For a review of this compelling documentary, see Travis Reimer, 'Christian Corner,' *Schizophrenia Digest* 1 (October 1994), 30–1.

29 Norman Cameron, 'Reason, Regression and Communication in Schizophren-

ics,' in *Pyschological Monographs*, Vol. 50, edited by John F. Dashiell (Columbus, OH: American Psychological Association 1938), 6.

30 'Caring is the antithesis of simply using the other person to satisfy one's own
needs' (Milton Mayeroff, *On Caring* [New York: Harper & Row 1971], 1).

31 See Parsons's *The Structure of Social Action* for a thorough critique of this dis-
tinguishing feature of conventional sociological inquiry.

32 Vygotsky, *Thought and Language*, 13.

33 Talcott Parsons addresses this issue in *The Structure of Social Action* in his
analysis of Vilfredo Pareto's significance to the theory of action and the difference between logical and nonlogical action.

34 Vygotsky, *Thought and Language*, 20.

35 Ibid., 149. At another point, Vygotsky writes: 'The relation between thought
and word is a living process; thought is born through words. A word devoid
of thought is a dead thing, and a thought unembodied in words remains a
shadow' (ibid., 153).

36 Torrey, *Surviving Schizophrenia*, 71.

36 Recall what Vygotsky means by 'inner speech': 'Inner speech is not the interior aspect of external speech – it is a function in itself. It still remains speech,
i.e., thought connected with words. But while in external speech thought is
embodied in words, in inner speech words die as they bring forth thought.
Inner speech is to a large extent thinking in pure meanings. It is a dynamic,
shifting, unstable thing, fluttering between word and thought, the two more
or less stable, more or less firmly delineated components of verbal thought'
(*Thought and Language*, 149).

38 Rosenberg, 'A Symbolic Interactionalist View of Psychosis,' 296–7.

38 On this issue, Rosenberg backpedals and writes: 'There are genuine differences between schizophrenics and other people beyond subjection to social
labeling' (ibid., 299). What are these differences? How do these differences lie
beyond social labelling? Is it possible not only to identify but also to evaluate
whether these differences are genuine?

40 Rosenberg gives up territory that he ought to fight to retain. Jeffrey C. Alexander writes: 'The issue ... is not which level is determinate or which disci-
pline is 'right' but, rather, at what level a given life phenonomenon should be
explained' (*Action and Its Environments: Toward a New Synthesis* [New York:
Columbia University Press 1988], 302). Alexander's theorizing exemplifies
the maturity required if sociology *vis-à-vis* the medical and psychiatric professions is to make meaningful contributions to the sociological study of
schizophrenia.

41 Our discussion has led to important issues with respect to the philosophy of
social linguistics. Vygotsky writes: 'Deliberate avoidance of philosophy is

itself a philosophy, and one that may involve its proponents in many inconsistencies' (*Thought and Language*, 20). I have pursued the issues with a concern for how they inform an adequate sociology of schizophrenia, with a
concern for how they inform an adequate understanding of the language of
people afflicted with schizophrenia. As indicated, the avoidance of the philosophical issues involves sociological inquiry in troublesome inconsistencies.

CHAPTER FOUR

1 *Mental Illness and Psychology* (Berkeley: University of California Press 1987),
   45. When addressing the significance of postmodernism in sociological
   inquiry, for purposes of clarity and understanding, it is helpful to keep in
   mind that the founders of postmodernism – Michel Focault, Jacques Lacan,
   Jacques Derrida, and Jean Baudrillard – are all admirers of the ancient Sophists. Foucault, for instance, identifies positively with Callicles in Plato's *Gor-
   gias* and Thrasymachus in the *Republic*. He resents the 'reassuring dialectic'
   that Socrates employs to refute his ancient friends, and it is as if Foucault
   believed that, if he were himself to encounter someone like Socrates, he,
   unlike his ancient friends, would remain firm in his defence of sophistry and
   antipathy towards Platonic philosophy. Postmodernism is the serious revival
   and unabashed celebration of the Sophists' critique of philosophy. One reason that postmodernism is gaining a wide audience and winning many con-
   cessions in the academy and theoretical sociology is that few still admire the
   exemplary character of Socrates as dramatized in the Platonic dialogues.
      The analogy to the ancient Sophists for the critical understanding of post-
   modernism is useful in several ways: It suggests that the spiritual founders
   of postmodernism are those successful Sophists, like Protagoras, who vehemently maintained that 'man is the measure of all things'; it indicates that
   Socrates (to stay within the paradigm) is the precursor and early representa-
   tive of what is now referred to as 'modernist thought' – postmodernism's
   demolished foil – and it recommends that sociological theorists might do
   well to reread the Platonic dialogues so as to gain a more knowledgeable
   reserve towards the unresisted claims of postmodernism.
2 Alan Blum writes on the role of the pariah and its limit: 'The fraternal
   warmth of excluded persons – of pariahs – co-exists with a disinterest or lack
   of responsiblity for worldly things and so for what things must mean. The
   very warmth and fraternity of pariah people that we have historically come
   to admire and celebrate is, at the same time, uninfluenced by care for the
   world and for cultivating worldly things in their discursive forms. The limits
   of the pariah are shown in the fact that his desire to write the history of suf-

fering conflicts with his rejection of discourse. The pariah rejects discourse because discourse undermines the authority of fraternity and puts into question the privileged authority of the sufferer himself' ('Victim, Patient, Client, Pariah: Steps in the Self-Understanding of the Experience of Suffering and Affliction,' *Reflections: Canadian Journal of Visual Impairment* 1 [1982], 80). The passage can be read as a critique of postmodernism's uncritical embrace of the pariah's as the ultimate viewpoint.

3 Deleuze and Guattari write: 'A schizophrenic out for a walk is a better model than a neurotic lying on the analyst's couch' (*Anti-Oedipus: Capitalism and Schizophrenia* [Minneapolis: University of Minnesota Press 1983], 2). To cite another example, consider this statement: 'Artaud makes a shambles of psychiatry, precisely because he is schizophrenic and not because he is not. Artaud is the fulfillment of literature, precisely because he is schizophrenic and not because he is not' (ibid., 135).

4 Harry Stack Sullivan, of course, does not advocate the postmodern perspective; he was a physician engaged in clinical research in search for a cure of schizophrenia, a search that the postmodern perspective would itself characterize as vain. Still, Sullivan's formulation of schizophrenia as a human phenomenon resonates with the postmodern understanding.

5 Harry Stack Sullivan, 'The Language of Schizophrenia' in *Language and Thought in Schizophrenia*, edited by J.S. Kasanin (New York: W.W. Norton 1964), 13.

6 George Herbert Mead, *Mind, Self, and Society* (Chicago: University of Chicago Press 1934), 175 and 178.

7 Ibid., 175

8 Ibid., 177–8.

9 Ibid., 178.

10 Louis A. Sass, *Madness and Modernism: Insanity in the Light of Modern Art, Literature, and Thought* (New York: Basic Books 1992), 133.

11 R.D. Laing, *The Divided Self* (Harmondsworth: Penguin 1969), 172. Compare Laing's comment on insight with Torrey's – 'Even in the stage of chronic illness an occasional person with schizophrenia will exhibit surprising insight' (E. Fuller Torrey, *Surviving Schizophrenia: A Family Manual*, rev. ed. [New York: Harper & Row 1988], 65); Laing and Torrey make the same observation but from different perspectives and with different understandings of what 'insight' means. Laing understands insight in an Hegelian sense, as a dialectical understanding and achievement on the part of self; Torrey understands insight in an empirical sense, as an objective observation that is hardly more than a matter of sense-perception.

12 For evidence of this point, consider this passage from Michel Foucault: 'The

critical ontology of ourselves has to be considered not, certainly, as a theory, a doctrine, nor even as a permanent body of knowledge that is accumulating; it has to be conceived as an attitude, an *ethos,* a philosophical life in which the critique of what we are is at one and the same time the historical analysis of the limits that are imposed on us and an experiment with the possibility of going beyond them' ('What Is Enlightenment?,' in *Interpretive Social Science: A Second Look,* edited by Paul Rabinow and William M. Sullivan [Berkeley: University of California Press 1987], 174).

What is Foucault saying? All that matters to ourselves is ourselves; nothing – no theory, no doctrine, no body of knowledge – exists to which we are subject, and this truth, according to Foucault, is the truth to which we are all subject. There is no reason to take the role of tradition, that is, 'the generalized other' that is culture. We ourselves are truth, and no other truth than ourselves exists.

13 Deleuze and Guattari, *Anti-Oedipus,* 361–2.
14 This Meadian formulation of Deleuze and Guattari's position is evident in the following passage: 'The task of schizoanalysis is that of tirelessly taking apart egos and their presuppositions; liberating the prepersonal singularities they enclose and repress [the work of self's 'I']; mobilizing the lows they would be capable of transmitting, receiving, or intercepting; establishing always further and more sharply the schizzes and the breaks well below conditions of identity ['I' detached from 'me']; and assembling the desiring-machines that countersect everyone and group everyone with others [society as a collection of 'I's, that is, 'non-me's]' (ibid, 362).
15 Ibid., 84.
16 Ibid., 360.
17 Foucault speaks against the idea of health as a metaphysical 'a priori' for social understanding. In postmodern theorizing, no Form, for instance, the Form of the Good, is said to exist. In a sense, Foucault is the ultimate positivist: 'Beyond mental pathology and organic pathology, there is a general, abstract pathology that dominates them both, imposing on them like so many prejudices, the same concepts and laying down for them, like so many postulates, the same methods. I would like to show that the root of mental pathology must be sought not in some kind of 'metapathology,' but in a certain relation, historically situated, of man to the madman and to the true man' (*Mental Illness and Psychology,* 2).

To know the true man is to know the true man in terms of a certain relation which is historically situated rather than in terms of some metaknowledge. The critical question is: How is the postmodern assumption of a 'true' man not tied up some kind of 'metaknowledge'? If historically situated man is the measure, to measure with something other than the historically situated is to fail to measure. With postmodernism, the practices of measure, interpretation, understanding, and judgment remain, but in demented and grotesque forms, that is, simply as expressions of power. The best measure becomes the immeasurable, the best interpretation the non-interpretable, and the best judgment the one which feigns non-judgment.

18. Deleuze and Guattari write: 'We believe in desire as in the irrational of every form of rationality, and not because it is a lack, a thirst, or an aspiration, but because it is the production of desire: desire that produces – real-desire, or the real itself' (*Anti-Oedipus*, 379).

19 Ibid., 362.

20 Deleuze and Guattari write: 'The schizophrenic process, which is not an illness, not a "breakdown" but a "breakthrough," however distressing and adventurous: breaking through the wall or the limit separating us from desiring-production, causing the flows of desire to circulate' (ibid., 362).

21 Mead, *Mind, Self, and Society*, 182.

22 Jorge Luis Borges, 'Borges and I,' in *Dreamtigers*, translated by Mildred Boyer and Harold Morland (Austin: University of Texas Press, 1985), 51.

23 Ibid.

24 Ibid.

25 Ibid.

26 The postmodern epistemology is discussed and critiqued in *Meno* as well as other Platonic dialogues. For an example of the ineffable paradox, consider the following exchange between Meno and Socrates:

> MENO: But how will you look for something when you don't in the least know what it is? How on earth are you going to set up something you don't know as the object of your search? To put it another way, even if you come right up against it, how will you know that what you have found is the thing you didn't know?
> SOCRATES: I know what you mean (Plato, *Protagoras and Meno* [Harmondsworth: Penguin 1956], 128).

27 Louis A. Sass writes in *Madness and Modernism*: 'It is ironic ... that the schizophrenic loss of self should have been taken, in antipsychiatry and in the artistic avant-garde, as some sign of liberation into the free play of desire. Actually, some such patients gradually cease to have any sexual feelings at all' (237).

28 Deleuze and Guattari confess as if their confession is no confession at all: 'Someone asked us if we had ever seen a schizophrenic – no, no, we have never seen one' (*Anti-Oedipus*, 380). For Deleuze and Guattari there is really

nothing to 'see'; what is to be seen is simply that there is no thing or idea, in and of itself, to be seen that can be called schizophrenia.

29 As Louis A. Sass points out in *Madness and Modernism*: 'Artaud did desire to eclipse the mind through ecstatic sensation and fusion with the ambient world; yet far from being his primordial condition, this was an escape he never achieved – not through drugs, not through the theatre of cruelty, not even through his own quest for the primitive, his famous voyage to the land of the Tarahumara Indians of Mexico (where he expected to find the world 'in

voyage to Mexico, he is profoundly disillusioned with his experiment in primitivism, his attempt to "liberate" his body by participating in the peyote rituals of the Tarahumara Indians. Now he can only marvel at "what false presentiment, what illusory and artificial intuition" could ever have given him these hopes' (239).

30 Notice the embarrassment in claiming to have been misunderstood, in claiming that self had been violated by another. On what basis would the postmodern theorist make this claim? Why would a postmodern theorist care unless self was in some sense constituted by a 'me'?

31 Deleuze and Guattari, *Anti-Oedipus*, 5.

32 Ibid., 380.

33 Sass writes: 'The literary *mise en abyme* has been described as a paradoxical combination of self-constitution and self-cancellation, a process in which categories are "torn apart" by their own self-referentiality ... [the] frantic attempt to constitute the self actually undermines it' (*Madness and Modernism*, 238).

34 Lev Vygotsky, *Thought and Language* (Cambridge, MA: MIT Press 1962), 149.

35 Torrey, *Surviving Schizophrenia*, 222.

36 Susan Sheehan, *Is There No Place on Earth for Me?* (New York: Vintage Books, 1983), 199.

37 Ibid.

CHAPTER FIVE

1 *Rabelais and His World* (Cambridge, MA: MIT Press 1968), 90–1.

2 Elaine Chaika, *Understanding Psychotic Speech: Beyond Freud and Chomsky* (Springfield, IL: Charles C. Thomas 1990), 31.

3 Louis A. Sass, *Madness and Modernism* (New York: Basic Books 1992), 152. Illogical thinking is defined as 'thinking that contains obvious internal contradictions or in which conclusions are reached that are clearly erroneous, given the initial premises.'

4 Kenneth Burke, *Perspectives by Incongruity* (Bloomington: Indiana University Press 1964), 94–5.

5 Roland Barthes writes: 'For what we grasp is not at all one term after the other, but the correlation which unites them: there are, therefore, the signifier, the signified, and the sign, which is the associative total of the first two terms' (*Mythologies*, translated by Annette Lavers, [New York: Noonday Press 1972], 113).

6 Chaika, *Understanding Psychotic Speech*, 296.

7 They invite analysis where the guiding assumption of such analysis is that language is dialogical. Bakhtin writes: 'When studying "dialogic speech," linguistics must utilize the results of metalinguistics. Dialogic relationships ... are extralinguistic. Language lives only in the dialogic interaction of those who make use of it. Dialogic interaction is indeed the authentic sphere where language *lives*' (*Problems of Dostoevsky's Poetics*, edited and translated by Caryl Emerson [Minneapolis: University of Minnesota Press 1983], 183).

8 Erving Goffman describes such a process as 'the betrayal funnel' in his essay 'The Moral Career of the Mental Patient,' in *Asylums* (Garden City, NY: Anchor Books 1961), 125–70. Goffman's title is itself a pun in that, given the cynical interactions that he describes, the title should be 'The Amoral Career of the Mental Patient.'

9 See Thomas Scheff on residual deviance in *Being Mentally Ill*, 2d ed. (New York: Aldine 1984).

10 We study puns as 'discourse, that is, language in its concrete living totality, and not language as the specific object of linguistics, something arrived at through a completely legitimate and necessary abstraction from various aspects of the concrete life of the word' (Bakhtin, *Problems of Dostoevsky's Poetics*, 181). 'The analyses that follow are not linguistic in the strict sense of the term. They belong rather to metalinguistics, if we understand by that term the study of those aspects in the life of the word, not yet shaped into separate and specific disciplines' (ibid.).

11 Paul Thibault, 'Paronomasia in Nabokov's *Ada*,' *Newcastle University Linguistic Students Journal* 4 (1978), 50.

12 Burke, *Perspectives by Incongruity*, 95.

13 An issue upon which I am not even touching is what would it mean for somone with schizophrenia to read this church sign. Would a person with schizophrenia experience the same thoughts that I am articulating here?

14 David E. Forrest does a comparable type of analysis of the poetry of e.e. cummings ('Nonsense and Sense in Schizophrenic Language,' *Schizophrenia Bulletin* 2 (1976), 286–301). Gilles Deleuze would call what Forrest is doing *qua*

literary criticism as well as this study *qua* semiology 'bad psychoanalysis'; 'Bad psychoanalysis has two ways of deceiving itself: it can believe that it has discovered identical subject matters, which necessarily can be found everywhere, or it can believe that it has found analogous forms which create false differences' ('The Schizophrenic and Language: Surface and Depth in Lewis Carroll and Antonin Artaud,' in *Textual Strategies: Perspectives in Post-Structualist Criticism*, edited by Josue V. Harari [Ithaca, NY: Cornell University Press 1979], 293).

15 The foundation for the inclusion for which this study argues is the notion of inner speech as formulated in Lev Vygotsky's *Thought and Language* (Cambridge, MA: MIT Press 1962). As argued in the previous chapter, there is no genuine or radical difference between people with schizophrenia and people without schizophrenia in that inner speech remains the source of thought, indeed thought itself, for people in both categories.

16 If a person with schizophrenia read this sign, what would be the person's reaction? Much as Piaget shows that children communicate better with adults than with each other, people with schizophrenia communicate better with people not afflicted with schizophrenia. Schizophrenic language and behaviour cannot be simulated as a way to reach out to people with schizophrenia any more than adults can use baby talk to reach out to young children. The question is: What is it for someone with schizophrenia to encounter 'normal' talk that has a 'schizophrenic' nature?

17 Chaika, *Understanding Psychotic Speech*, 13.

18 See Dianne F. Herman, 'The Rape Culture,' in *Women: A Feminist Perspective*, edited by Jo Freeman (Mountain View, CA: Mayfield 1984).

19 Chaika, *Understanding Psychotic Speech*, 6.

20 Ibid, 212.

21 Hugo Meynell descibes the issue and the perspective which this study advocates *vis-à-vis* Chaika's work with the following comment: 'We may distinguish, then, between two fundamental kinds of influence on the behavior of an agent: (a) that which treats him *as an agent* in the kinds of way that I have just described, and (b) that which affects him by means such as one might apply to an inanimate object, plant, or lower animal. One of the central points at issue between Laing and his opponents is whether schizophrenic patients ought to be treated in the first kind of way – as agents, by the methods of persuasion customarily used upon agents – or in the second kind of way, which does not take into account their status as agents' ('Philosophy and Schizophrenia,' *Journal of the British Society for Phenomenology* 2 [1971], 20).

22 Here is a another example of someone taking the position which is being opposed: 'The sentences – "I have many ties with my home. My father wears

them around his collar" – seem to skip, like a stone on a lake, from *ties* (bonds) to *home* to *father* to *ties* (neckties). On the surface, this is a witty statement, but the speaker had no idea of what was really going on inside or underneath the form of words. The statement was therefore unwitting and hence unwitty' (Brendan A. Maher in *Psychology Today*, November 1968, 60. The point of this chapter is to dissuade readers from jumping to Maher's particular conclusion.

23 Vygotsky, *Thought and Language*, 126.

24 Chaika herself suggests this anterior notion when she writes: 'One thing to note ... is that each of the fragments can be restored by English speaking hearers ... No one needs training in this skill. It comes from beng a human being who has learned a language. This is what is meant by "normal decoding strategy"' (*Understanding Psychotic Speech*, 289).

25 Gregory Bateson, 'Toward a Theory of Schizophrenia,' with Don D. Jackson, Jay Haley, and John Weakland, in *Steps to an Ecology of Mind: Collected Essays in Anthropology, Psychiatry, Evolution, and Epistemology* by Gregory Bateson (San Francisco: Chadler 1972), 225.

26 At first blush it does not seem that the example can be analysed because we only know what Bateson tells us and because we are not certain whether this obedient patient has schizophrenia. Nevertheless, given Bateson's commitment and the behaviour described, we can deduce that, for the author, this behaviour is an instance of literalness, the inability to distinguish between the concrete and the metaphoric. If that is the case, from Bateson's psychoanalytic point of view, it does become an example of schizophrenic behaviour.

27 Harold Searles writes: 'It gradually became apparent to me that his literal mode of thought, serving as an unconscious defense against a welter of repressed affects, was a product of the tenuousness of his ego boundaries' ('The Differentiation between Concrete and Metaphorical Thinking in the Recovering Schizophrenic Patient,' in *Collected Papers on Schizophrenia and Related Subjects* [New York: International Universities Press 1965], 565).

28 Max Weber, *The Theory of Social and Economic Organization* (New York: Free Press 1947), 112.

29 Searles writes: 'I had worked with schizophrenic patients for several years before I came to realize that the deeply schizophrenic individual has, subjectively, no imagination' (*The Differentiation between Concrete and Metaphorical Thinking,'* 574).

30 Bakhtin, *Rabelais and His World*, 49, and Bakhtin cited in Michael Gardiner, *The Dialogics of Critique: M.M. Bakhtin and the Theory of Ideology* (London: Routledge 1992), 48. Gardiner provides an excellent introduction to the corpus of Bakhtin's work and its compelling significance to sociological inquiry.

31 Michel Foucault, *Madness and Civilization: A History of Insanity in the Age of Reason* (New York: Vantage Books 1973), 33.

32 Bakhtin writes: 'The principle of laughter and the carnival spirit on which grotesque is based destroys this limited seriousness and all pretense of an extratemporal meaning and unconditional value of necessity. It frees human consciousness, thought, and imagination for new potentialities' (*Rabelais and His World*, 49).

33 Jean-Paul Sartre, *Anti-Semite and Jew*, translated by George J. Becker (New York: Schocken Books 1965), 20.

34 Foucault, *Madness and Civilization*, 27.

CHAPTER SIX

1 *Thought and Language*, translation newly revised and edited by Alex Kozulin (Cambridge, MA: MIT Press 1986), 252. This later edition includes a sentence that the earlier one did not: 'Thought is not the superior authority in the process.' It is interesting that in the earlier translation the editor censored this statement.

2 Max Weber, *The Theory of Social and Economic Organization* (New York: Oxford University Press 1947), 99.

3 The writing of Oliver Sacks is animated in eloquent ways by this issue of how the mind functions independently from the brain. That is, while Sacks writes from a neurological point of view, he often finds himself on metaphysical turf.

4 Talcott Parsons states the point in the following way: 'Whatever the importance of neurological prerequisites may be, it seems probable that true symbolization as distinguished from the use of signs, cannot arise or function without the interaction of actors, and that the individual actor can acquire symbolic systems only through interaction with social objects' (*The Social System* [New York: Free Press 1951], 10).

5 Charles Cooley writes: 'By human nature, I suppose, we may understand those sentiments and impulses that are human in being superior to those of lower animals ... particularly, sympathy and the innumerable sentiments into which sympathy enters, such as love, resentment, ambition, vanity, hero-worship, and the feeling of social right and wrong' (*Social Organization: A Study of the Larger Mind* [New York: Schocken Books 1962], 28).

6 Nancy Andreason, *The Broken Brain: The Biological Revolution in Psychiatry* (New York: Harper & Row 1984), 253.

7 There is a much funding for neurological and genetic research on schizophrenia because schizophrenia provides the natural sciences with the opportu-

nity to address that part of the human brain that is absent from the brains of other members of the animal kingdom. Schizophrenia offers the natural sciences the opportunity to address what is unique in nature about the human species and, in so doing, perhaps influence the very course and development of the human species. The natural sciences, in other words, like all action, are governed by motivation as much as by thought. Science, in other words, is subject to sociological analysis.

8 Weber writes: 'In order to give a precise meaning to these terms, it is necessary for the sociologist to formulate pure ideal types of the corresponding forms of action which in each case involve the highest possible degree of logical integration by virtue of their complete adequacy on the level of meaning' (*The Theory of Social and Economic Organization*, 110).

9 What is the epistemological foundation of the ideal type? The issue is a difficult one. As Weber writes: 'In no case does it [the theoretically conceived *pure type* of subjective meaning attributed to the hypothetical actor or actors in a given type of action] refer to an objectively "correct" meaning or one which is "true" in some metaphysical sense' (ibid., 89).

   If sociology does not seek to ascertain the 'true' and 'valid' meanings associated with the objects of its investigation, what then does sociology seek to ascertain? How is the meaningfulness of 'the theoretically conceived *pure types* of subjective meaning' that Weber seeks to ascertain distinct from the 'true' and 'valid' meanings associated with the objects of their investigation? How is it that only the ideal type can put the sociologist in touch with this ontology? How important is this ontology to the development of sociological knowledge? How is this ontology, that is central to the development of sociological knowledge, distinct from a Utopia-like knowledge? How is it real? There is a vast amount of Weberian scholarship that addresses but does not answer these questions.

10 Talcott Parsons, *The Structure of Social Action* (New York: Free Press 1968), 603.

11 R.D. Laing, *The Divided Self* (Harmondsworth: Penguin 1969), 9.

12 Laing's goal is to show how one cannot hear the person with schizophrenia when one's interest is simply to measure and test the person as an organic thing. Laing brings this point to our attention forcefully when he analyses the transcript of Emil Kraepelin's interview of a schizophrenic patient in a lecture hall: 'This patient's behavior can be seen in at least two ways ... One may see his behavior as "signs" of a "disease"; one may see his behavior as expressive of his existence ... What is the boy's experience of Kraepelin? He seems to be tormented and desperate. What is he "about" in speaking and acting in this way? He is objecting to being measured and tested. He wants to

be heard' (ibid., 30–1). Kraepelin discovers no law for the relation of the subject's self-consciousness to his actuality. Kraepelin obstructs such an understanding. G.W.F. Hegel articulates this problem as the limit of observation as an instance of authentic understanding: 'Psychological observation discovers no law for the relation of self-consciousness to actuality' (*The Phenomenology of Mind*, translated by J.B. Baille [Atlantic Highlands, NJ: Humanities Press 1977], 338).

13 E. Fuller Torrey, *Surviving Schizophrenia: A Family Manual*, rev. ed. (New York: Harper & Row 1988), 166.

14 Ibid.

15 Charging reification is not uncommon in the social sciences. The philosopher Morris Raphael Cohen provides a good account of the way in which Torrey employs the term. Cohen uses reification to chastise any work that neglects positivism as the unconditional foundation for the development of scientific research. Here is an example that pertains to psychology: 'In thus rejecting the soul as the subject-matter of science of psychology, we do not discriminate against any known phase of conscious life. But we set ourselves against the fallacy of reification, of supposing that because we can speak of the soul as a noun or subject of discourse it must necessarily be an existing thing in which properties inhere. This fallacy of reification is not avoided if for the word *soul* we substitute any other term such as the *consciousness* or *unconscious mind*, the *non-empirical self, the psychic organism independent of the body*, or the like. Conscious life is a series of events in the history of an organism. It is not a separate non-empirical thing' (Morris Cohen, *Reason and Nature* [New York: Dover Publications 1978], 302). For Cohen, psychology must dismiss the notion of soul (and any of its contemporary euphemisms such as 'conscious' or 'unconscious' mind) as signifying a significant ontology for the understanding of the human being. The notion of soul, Cohen says, is too metaphysical and mythological for science to take at all seriously. The power of Cohen's statement ('Power consists in the ability to restrict and limit meaning' (J.F. MacCannell, *Figuring Lacan – Criticism and the Cultural Unconscious* [Lincoln: University of Nebraska Press 1986], 47) is the way in which it cuts off escape from the conclusions of positivism. Cohen asserts that, after dismissing the notion of soul as a meaningful ontology for understanding the human being, psychology cannot compensate for what is now missing by substituting any concept that still hints at the existence of a non-empirical self. For Cohen what is instead signified by such wishy-washy terms can be only that complex, human subject constituted as 'a series of events in the history of an organism.'

It is disappointing that, in a footnote to Weber's text, Parsons, as editor and translator, favourably cites Cohen's discussion of epistemology as enhancing Weber's discussion of theory construction in the social sciences (see Weber, *The Theory of Social and Economic Organization*, 103). Weber does not actually advocate the epistemology that Cohen does. More strongly, Weber frees sociological theorists from the need to work within the constraints that Cohen recommends. Weber says that, to study the human being as a social actor, sociologists draw upon a degree of knowledge that cannot itself be controlled by a positivistic epistemology. Parsons's citation of Cohen derails Weber's key point.

16 Burke Thomason defines reification this way: '"Reification" can be understood as a cognitive process whereby various aspects of experience come to acquire a kind of inappropriate ontological fixedness' (*Making Sense of Reification: Alfred Schutz and Constructionist Theory* [Atlantic Highlands, NJ: Humanities Press 1982], 88).

17 Weber, *The Theory of Social and Economic Organization*, 110.

18 Ibid.

19 R.W. Comstock, 'Hegel, Kierkegaard, Marx on "The Unhappy Consciousness",' *Int. Jahrbuck fur Wissens und Religions Soziologie* 11 (1978), 96.

20 A first-person account cited by Brendan A. Maher in *Psychology Today,* November 1968, 33.

21 Stanley Rosen, *G.W.F. Hegel* (New Haven: Yale University Press 1974), 151.

22 Ibid., 152.

23 Consider this passage from Hegel and how it could stand as a description of the self-consciousness of someone with schizophrenia: 'This unhappy consciousness, divided and at variance within itself, must, because this contradiction of its essential nature is felt to be a single consciousness, always have in the one consciousness the other also; and thus must be straightway driven out of each in turn, when it thinks it has therein attained to the victory and rest of unity' (*The Phenomenology of Mind*, 251).

24 Laing is influenced by Jean-Paul Sartre's analysis of bad faith. Bad faith is, in fact, Sartre's reworking the Hegelian concept of the Unhappy Consciousness. Thus, Laing is influenced by Hegel's formulation of the Unhappy Consciousness through Sartre's understanding of the Unhappy Consciousness as formulated in Sartre's account of bad faith (see Sartre, referenced in Laing, *The Divided Self*, 95–6).

It should be noted that, at times, Laing employs the Unhappy Consciousness to explicate the subjective meaningfulness of disorders other than schizophrenia, for instance, hysteria. While, from a positivistic point of view, this tendency may seem frustrating, from the point of view of this study, it is reassuring. While not empiricially coherent, Laing at least is conceptually coherent. Laing's reification occurs because Laing is fixated on the concept of the Unhappy Consciousness as a therapist and an intellectual.

25 Hegel writes: 'Stoicism, therefore, got embarrassed when, as the expression went, it was asked for the criterion of truth in general, i.e., properly speaking, for a content of thought itself' (*The Phenomenology of Mind*, 246). The Stoic got embarrassed because the Stoic is unable to account for the determinateness of its pure thought.

26 'In Skepticism,' Hegel says, 'the entire unessentiality and unsubstantiality of this "other" becomes a reality for consciousness' (ibid., 246).

27 Speaking of the principle that governs this discursive practice, Hegel states: 'If sameness is shown to it, it points out unlikeness, non-identity; and when the latter, which has expressly mentioned the moment before, is held up to it, it passes on to indicate sameness and identity' (ibid., 250).

28 Consider the following passage on the nature of the Unhappy Consciousness: 'Its thinking as such is no more than the discordant clang of ringing bells, or a cloud of warm incense, a kind of thinking in terms of music, that does not get the length of notions, which would be the sole, immanent, objective mode of thought. This boundless pure inward feeling comes to have indeed its object; but this object does not make its appearance in conceptual form, and therefore comes on the scene as something external and foreign' (ibid., 257). The widely accepted exegesis of this passage is that it discloses Hegel's critique of the pious consciousness. The passage introduces Hegel's philosophy of religion, where medieval Christianity is the object of his analysis – 'the discordant clang of ringing bells, or a cloud of warm incense.' Rosen, to summarize as well as extend the different interpretive responses of Hegelian scholars to this text, writes: 'The unhappy consciousness surely has pagan, Jewish, and Christian forms, and modern as well as ancient variations' (*G.W.F. Hegel*, 169). The achievement of Laing's work is his formulation of schizophrenia as a concrete variation and reified form of the Unhappy Consciousness.

For example, what does it mean to think and speak without getting to 'the length of notions, which would be the sole, immanent, objective mode of thought'? What is this 'kind of thinking in terms of music,' which 'comes to have indeed its object; but this object does not make its appearance in conceptual form, and therefore comes on the scene as something external and foreign'? Yes, Hegel is thinking of a certain kind of religiosity, but the passage can also be employed as an ideal type to enlarge the parameters of social epistemology through which, at an explanatory level, we may account for the self-consciousness of someone with schizophrenia.

29 Hegel, *The Phenomenology of Mind*, 663.

30 Sylvia Nasar, 'The Lost Years of a Nobel Laureate,' *The New York Times*, Business Section, 13 November 1994.
31 Ibid.
32 Hegel writes: 'This unity of objectivity and independent self-existence which lies in the notion of action, and which therefore comes for consciousness to be the essential reality and object – as this is not taken by consciousness to be the principle of its action, neither does it become an object for consciousness directly and through itself' (*The Phenomenology of Mind*, 267).
33 Laing cites the *Phenomenology* only once in *The Divided Self*, and the citation is a passage that occurs well after Hegel's analysis of the Unhappy Consciousness. If Laing cites Hegel only once, and the passage he cites is not from the section on the Unhappy Consciousness, how can it be argued that Laing employs this notion as an ideal type in his account of schizophrenia?

The passage which Laing cites is on the essence of action: 'The act is something simple, determinate, universal, to be grasped as an abstract, distinctive whole; it is murder, theft, a benefit, a deed of bravery, and so on, and what it *is* can be *said* of it. It *is* such, and such, and its being is not merely a symbol, it is the fact itself' (Hegel, cited in *The Divided Self*, 87). This passage represents the anterior idea to Hegel's discussion of the Unhappy Consciousness. The Unhappy Consciousness abhors action (what 'is simple, determinate, universal,
the action of the Unhappy Consciousness. Laing appreciates that the crucial point in Hegel's analysis of the Unhappy Consciousness is the one which the Unhappy Consciousness suppresses and which comes to full light only later in the *Phenomenology*.

EPILOGUE

1 'Victim, Patient, Client, Pariah: Steps in the Self-Understanding of Suffering and Affliction,' *Reflections: Canadian Journal of Visual Impairment* 1 (1982), 65.
2 *The Structure of Social Action* (New York: Free Press 1968), 162.
3 'A fact is referred to as "an empirically verifiable *statement* about phenomena." The point is that a fact is not itself a phenomenon at all, but a proposition *about* one or more phenomena' (ibid., 41).
4 This talk was published under the title 'Volunteering' in *Schizophrenia Digest*, 2/2 (1995), 14–15.

Index